18 3 00

Auditory Processing and Language

Authors are listed alphabetically.
Christine Sloan formerly published as Christine Harris.

Auditory Processing and Language
Clinical and Research Perspectives

edited by

Philip J. Levinson, Ph.D.

Director, Scottish Rite Institute for Childhood Aphasia
Portland, Oregon
formerly *University Affiliated Program*
Childrens Hospital of Los Angeles
and Department of Speech
University of California, Santa Barbara

Christine Sloan, Ph.D.

Boulder, Colorado
formerly, *Director, Hearing and Speech Clinic*
Childrens Hospital of Los Angeles

Grune & Stratton

A Subsidiary of Harcourt Brace Jovanovich, Publishers
New York London Toronto Sydney San Francisco

Grune & Stratton, Inc.
111 Fifth Avenue
New York, New York 10003

Distributed in the United Kingdom by
Academic Press, Inc. (London) Ltd.
24/28 Oval Road, London NW1

Library of Congress Catalog Number 80-83870
International Standard Book Number 0-8089-1305-0
Printed in the United States of America

*To Beth, Noel, and all the other children
who were our inspiration and teachers.*

Contents

Special Acknowledgment

Three of the contributors to this volume studied under the direction of Hildred Schuell, a leader in adult aphasia, who was associated with the Veterans Hospital and University of Minnesota Hospitals, Minneapolis. Her memory continues to provide an inspiration to her students. She was a careful observer of behavior and possessed a genuine curiosity about the human mind and its capacity for communication. With this attitude she believed she could come to understand her patients directly, without preconceptions. She admonished her students, *let the patient teach you*. For many of us this was the most valuable advice ever given. We acknowledge her inspiration and the example she set forth of professional expertise and integrity.

Christine Sloan
Boulder, Colorado
April 1980

Preface

This book grew out of a conference on the clinical application of research in auditory processing held at Childrens Hospital of Los Angeles in April, 1977. The objective of the conference was to present current research in the area of auditory processing and to discuss its applicability to clinical populations and clinical methods. What developed from that meeting was an awareness that there is all too little communication between persons in the clinical and research areas. There seemed to be a need to bring information from both of these professional spheres together so that each may benefit. It seemed important for clinicians to carefully examine the methods and results of research, and then to apply and test these as part of the clinical process. On the other hand, it seemed equally important for researchers to know the data on clinical populations and treatment procedures that clinicians were collecting—the individual differences and patterns of behavior that presented themselves in the clinical setting. Clinical information of this nature can often guide and focus research investigations.

The individuals contributing to this volume seem to have an interest and commitment to this kind of communication between research and clinical application, each from a particular perspective and area of interest. All of these authors have in common an interest in auditory perception and the processes that relate this to speech and language.

Robert Stillman has been in neurophysiologic research and more recently specialized in electrophysiologic measures of auditory function; however, he has also been a keen observer of behavior, and has developed observational scales of behavior such as the Callier-Azusa Scale, designed to aid in the assessment of deaf-blind and severely handicapped children. He has been interested in the clinical application of research and in correlating clinical findings with research results.

Patricia Kuhl has had a varied research background that includes studies of clinical populations, highly specific psychoacoustic research, animal research, and most recently investigations of infant speech perception. In addition, she trained as a clinical speech pathologist and has had clinical experience in both childhood and adult language disorders. Like Paula Tallal, she has contributed significantly to our understanding of speech processing in young infants, not only in terms of the results of her investigations, but also in terms of the methods of investigation that she developed. These methods have relevance for both the research and clinical fields.

Paula Tallal has accomplished one of the most significant investigations of auditory processing in a clinical population. She developed a research methodology that begins to separate the contributions of perceptual and linguistic factors in auditory processing. Her work exemplifies a clinical approach transformed into a reliable research methodology. It is of benefit in both research and clinical spheres. In addition, it is significant in that she demonstrated how one group of subjects can be studied in a thorough and systematic way.

Marie Poulsen and Philip Levinson bring together the perspectives of two disciplines in relating a theory of cognitive development to the varied observations and studies of auditory behavior in very early childhood. This integration provides a framework for both clinical and research investigations. These authors have observed the behavior of many young children, and have developed together an interdisciplinary view of child development and the role of auditory processing within that framework.

Christine Sloan has worked clinically with both children and adults with language disorders. She worked for several years with Hildred Schuell, and investigated the auditory perceptual problems of adult aphasic patients. Her more recent work with children has been devoted to understanding the underlying processes that are impaired in children with language disorders, and in documenting methods of treatment that are effective. She emphasizes that the same precision and specificity one finds in research methodologies can be applied in the clinical process. The clinican can "field test" the results of research and either substantiate or disclaim these findings.

Kathleen Johnston worked closely with Hildred Schuell in adult aphasia for many years as clinician and research investigator, a role she continues in the Department of Neurology at the University of Minnesota. She exemplifies the ongoing relationship that is needed between these two areas of inquiry. She is a keen observer of behavior and a careful and systematic investigator of the processes and conditions that produce it.

Isabelle Liberman, Donald Shankweiler, and their colleagues at the University of Connecticut were included in this volume for several reasons. Their work deals with higher language functions—reading and writing—and in this way provides the continuity that exists as one moves from infant speech perception to later reading achievement. Their research also exemplifies the approach of the entire volume. It is a "process" approach; they are interested in the processes that contribute to success in early reading instruction. Their investigations led to the discovery of the importance of phonologic factors in reading.

In general the contributors to this volume seem to view language and language processes quite broadly. However, they represent an approach to understanding language that attempts to discover the individual components contributing to the total process. Language is a complex human activity. We have chosen to view this activity from a "process" perspective. We have put together a collection of chapters that elucidate the nature and role of one component of language behavior, auditory processing. We take the view that clinical and research perspectives share equally in contributing to our further understanding of this area of inquiry about language.

We would like to acknowledge the help and support of several people: Shirley Schrier, Hearing and Speech Division, Childrens Hospital of Los Angeles, for her support in assisting with the organization of the conference that led to this book, and for her suggestions about its development; Liz Dennon, for assisting with typing; Alan Sloan and Dianne Levinson, for their support and encouragement to continue what seemed like a never ending task; and finally, Emily Levinson, who, at what seemed like the busiest times, said, "Daddy, I need a hug."

Contributors

Benita Blachman, Ph.D.
School of Education
Syracuse University
Syracuse, New York
formerly, Department of Educational Psychology
University of Connecticut
Storrs, Connecticut

Linda Camp
Department of Educational Psychology
University of Connecticut
Storrs, Connecticut

Kathleen L. Johnston, B.A.
Department of Neurology
University of Minnesota Medical School
Minneapolis, Minnesota

Patricia K. Kuhl, Ph.D.
Department of Speech and Hearing Sciences
and
Child Development and Mental Retardation Center
University of Washington
Seattle, Washington

Philip J. Levinson, Ph.D.
Scottish Rite Institute for Childhood Aphasia
Portland, Oregon
formerly, University Affiliated Program

Childrens Hospital of Los Angeles
Los Angeles, California
and
Department of Speech
University of California, Santa Barbara
Santa Barbara, California

Isabelle Y. Liberman, Ph.D.
Department of Educational Psychology
University of Connecticut
Storrs, Connecticut
and
Haskins Laboratories
New Haven, Connecticut

Marie K. Poulsen, Ph.D.
University Affiliated Program
Childrens Hospital of Los Angeles
Los Angeles, California

Donald Shankweiler, Ph.D.
Department of Psychology
University of Connecticut
Storrs, Connecticut
and
Haskins Laboratories
New Haven, Connecticut

Christine Sloan, Ph.D.
(formerly published as Christine Harris)
Boulder, Colorado
formerly Director, Hearing and Speech Clinic
Childrens Hospital of Los Angeles
Los Angeles, California

Robert Stillman, Ph.D.
Program in Communication Disorders
University of Texas at Dallas
and
Callier Center for Communication Disorders
Dallas, Texas

Paula Tallal, Ph.D.
Department of Psychiatry
University of California, San Diego
La Jolla, California

Michele Werfelman
Department of Educational Psychology
University of Connecticut
Storrs, Connecticut

Auditory Processing and Language

Robert Stillman

1

Auditory Brain Mechanisms

The auditory system, like all sensory systems, evolved from the need of organisms to detect, locate, and identify consequential aspects of their environment. The auditory system differs from other sensory systems only in its specialization, the ability to respond to sounds emitted by vibrating structures in the environment.

The auditory system is made up of functionally distinct peripheral and central components. The peripheral components are uniquely designed to receive and transduce sound energy. They have evolved to maximize reception of consequential sounds, to do the initial analysis, and to transduce this information into the neuroelectric code of the brain. The central component operates entirely on neuroanatomic connections and neuroelectric codes. Its role is to extract from the acoustic array transduced at the periphery, the events vital to the organism's functioning.

EXTERNAL EAR AND EAR CANAL

The only auditory system components visible on the surface of the head are the external ear and the entrance to the ear canal. Other receptive structures, including the tympanic membrane, the ossicular chain, and the cochlea are, for protection, located deep within the head.

The external ear is primarily a sound collecting device. It gathers sound waves and directs them into the ear canal. In most species, the external ear is mobile in order to better subserve its sound collecting and directing function. In humans, the external ear is relatively small and, therefore, somewhat limited in its sound collecting ability. One may artificially extend the external ear by cupping the hand behind it and thereby obtain a slight improvement in hearing sensitivity.

Sound waves directed into the ear canal strike the tympanic membrane (eardrum), which seals the canal at its internal end. Some of the sound energy sets the tympanic membrane in motion. The remainder is reflected back toward the ear canal entrance. Due to the length of the ear canal, reflected sound energy in the 2 to 6 kHz frequency range resonates within the canal. The resonance intensifies sounds between 2 and 6 kHz and thereby increases the audibility of these sounds.

MIDDLE EAR

Vibration of the tympanic membrance activates the ossicular chain, three tiny serially connected bones. Through the ossicular chain, mechanical vibrations—faithfully replicating in frequency, amplitude, and duration the sounds which initiated them—are conducted to the cochlea. The first ossicle, the malleus, is attached at one end to the tympanic membrane. At the other end of the malleus, a relatively stiff joint connects the malleus to the second ossicle, the incus. Under normal circumstances, malleus movement is transmitted undistorted to the incus. The incus connects to the third ossicle, the stapes, and the stapes connects to the oval window of the cochlea. Stapes vibrations are directly transmitted to the cochlear fluids through the oval window.

To assure freedom of movement, the ossicles are suspended by ligaments within a hollow, air-filled space—the middle ear cavity. Because the middle ear cavity is air-filled, a mechanism for air pressure equalization between inside and outside the head is provided. This mechanism, the eustachian tube, connects the middle ear cavity to the nasopharynx. The periodic movement of air through the eustachian tube equalizes pressure across the tympanic membrane, placing tension on it. This reduces the ability of the tympanic membrane to vibrate to sounds and decreases auditory sensitivity.

The transduction of sound waves into the mechanical vibration of the tympanic membrance and ossicles permits the efficient conversion of sound pressure to fluid pressure within the cochlea. In the absence of the tympanic membrane and ossicles, about 99.9 percent of the airborne sound energy would be reflected at the air/fluid interface, the oval window of the cochlea. To illustrate this problem, consider trying to speak to someone submerged in water. The sound pressure of your voice is transmitted to the listener only with considerable loss in intensity. Most of the airborne sound energy is reflected at the surface of the water. The role of the middle ear apparatus is to compensate for the energy loss at the air/fluid interface by mechanically increasing the force of vibrations delivered to the cochlear fluids. The boost in force is accomplished primarily by focusing the sound energy collected across the large surface area of the tympanic membrane on to the small oval window, the entrance to the cochlea. Leverage between the tympanic membrane and the malleus, and between the malleus and stapes (via the incus), accounts for a small additional gain in force.

The middle ear apparatus normally functions as a highly efficient transduction system. However, under certain circumstances to the organism's advantage, the mechanism automatically becomes inefficient. In the presence of intense sounds potentially damaging to the fragile cochlear structures, the joints between the malleus and incus, and between the stapes and oval window, partially disarticulate. This prevents the full force of malleus movement from reaching the cochlea.

Cochlear protection during intense acoustic stimulation also may be afforded by the acoustic reflex, the reflexive contraction of the middle ear muscles attached to the ossicular chain. There are two middle ear muscles: the tensor tympani attached to the malleus, and the stapedius attached to the stapes. These two muscles operate independently, or in concert, to stiffen the ossicular chain and reduce its amplitude of motion.

The acoustic reflex is initiated most readily by high-frequency sounds. However, because muscle contraction stiffens the ossicular chain, the reflex attenuates only low frequencies. In fact, transmission of 1 to 2 kHz vibrations is actually facilitated a few dB by muscle contraction, while transmission of lower frequencies is substantially attenuated.[1] The important role of the acoustic reflex, however, is not cochlear protection but the improvement of signal-to-noise ratio. This is accomplished by the selective attenuation of moderate and intense low-frequency sounds (noise) when they co-occur with sounds of higher frequency, typically most consequential for the organism.

The selective attenuation of low-frequency sounds by the middle ear muscles is necessary because intense low frequencies readily mask or decrease the audibility of simultaneously present high frequencies. Since consequential complex sounds such as vocalizations and speech are often discriminable only by their high-frequency components, it is important that the low-frequency components of these sounds do not interfere with the perception of the high-frequency components. The role of the middle-ear muscles in improving signal-to-noise ratio can be demonstrated in individuals with inoperative middle ear muscles. Such individuals have difficulty discriminating intense speech, but not speech below the level of the acoustic reflex threshold.[2] The perceptual difficulty of these individuals is related to the fact that, at higher stimulus intensity levels, the low-frequency components of speech mask perception of the higher frequency features necessary for accurate discrimination.

Reflex contraction of the middle ear muscles does not always require the presence of an external sound. Internal activities that generate noise such as chewing, swallowing, startle responses, and vocalizations also activate the middle ear muscles. Furthermore, they do this independently of the sound's intensity and sometimes prior to the sound's occurrence.[2] It appears that the middle ear muscles function to reduce the masking effect of low-frequency sounds, in this case internal noise. This mechanism then, allows the organism to retain sensitivity to consequential high-frequency sounds while engaging in activities that generate potentially masking low-frequency noise.

COCHLEAR MECHANICS

The transduction of sound-initiated mechanical vibrations into neuroelectric codes for transmission to the brain takes place in the cochlea. Structurally, the cochlea is a bony, coiled tube similar in shape to a snail shell. The base of the cochlea is exposed to the middle ear cavity, and the apex or termination of the cochlea is buried within the temporal bone. Inside the cochlea are three fluid-filled chambers. Each runs the length of the cochlea from base to apex. The middle chamber, the cochlear partition, is totally enclosed. The cochlear partition includes the scala media and is separated from the upper chamber (scala vestibuli) by Reissner's membrane and from the lower chamber (scala tympani) by the basilar membrane. Resting on the basilar membrane is the Organ of Corti. The Organ of Corti contains the auditory receptor cells which convert mechanical vibrations to electrical activity.

The fluid-filled chambers of the cochlea are sealed in bone except for two small membrane-covered openings, the oval and the round windows. Both openings are at the base of the cochlea and are exposed to the middle ear cavity. The footplate of the stapes fits over the oval window so that sound-initiated ossicular vibrations directly affect the fluid of the scala vestibuli. The round window, in the scala tympani, opens unimpeded into the middle ear cavity.

Except for the oval and the round windows, the cochlea is functionally sealed. Positive and negative fluid pressure that builds up in the cochlea following inward and outward stapes movement can be relieved only by outward and inward movement of the round window membrane. Pressure in the scala vestibuli following stapes movement is transferred to the scala tympani through the flexible cochlear partition. For frequencies within the audible range, the build-up of fluid pressure in the scala vestibuli during inward stapes movement depresses the cochlear partition which, in turn, forces the fluid of the scala tympani against the round window. The flexibility of the cochlear partition is not equal from apex to base. Rather, its flexibility is graded such that it is most flexible at the apex and becomes progressively stiffer toward the base. von Békésy, in his classic studies of cochlear mechanics, demonstrated that the graded flexibility of the cochlear partition results in an orderly or tonotopic relationship between the stimulus frequency and the region of the cochlear partition displaced.[3] Low-frequency sounds maximally displace the most apical regions and progressively higher frequency sounds affect progressively more basal regions. Each stimulus frequency, therefore, maximally displaces a distinct region of the cochlear partition and the region displaced is directly related to the stimulus frequency.

Although the region of maximal displacement along the cochlear partition is fixed for each frequency, the length of the cochlear partition displaced and the amplitude of displacement is a function of sound intensity (amplitude of stapes movement). Thus, a suprathreshold sound of 500 Hz vibrates the cochlear partition at 500 Hz not only in the region most sensitive to 500 Hz, but also in adjacent regions—regions most sensitive to frequencies above and below 500 Hz. The amplitude of displacement of the cochlear partition at any point is directly related to the intensity of the stimulus.

The area of the cochlear partition displaced by suprathreshold tones is asymmetrically distributed around the region of maximum sensitivity. A much greater length is displaced basally than apically from the region of maximal displacement. The spread of low-frequency vibrations to more basal cochlear regions results in the usurpation by intense low frequencies of regions of the cochlear partition normally sensitive to higher frequencies. This explains why intense low-frequency sounds interfere with or mask the perception of less intense sounds of higher frequency. The role of the middle ear muscles in the improvement of the signal-to-noise ratio is accomplished by the reduction in amplitude of low frequencies delivered to the cochlea. This reduces the basal spread of low-frequency vibration along the cochlear partition, and allows the more basal regions to retain their sensitivity to simultaneously occurring high-frequency sounds.

The displacement of the cochlear partition over time takes the form of a traveling wave. For suprathreshold sounds, the basal region is displaced first, followed by successively more apical regions up to and just beyond the point of maximal displacement for the particular stimulus frequency. Each point on the cochlear partition responds with a characteristic time delay following stapes movement; this delay is independent of the frequency or intensity of the sound. Basal cochlear regions are activated almost instantly by stapes movement while the most apical regions do not respond until almost 5 msec later.

The cochlear partition carries out the initial analysis of sound frequency and intensity. The next step is the conversion of mechanical action at each point on the cochlear partition into electrical activity for transmission to the brain.

MECHANICAL TO ELECTRICAL TRANSDUCTION IN THE COCHLEA

The transduction of acoustic information from mechanical to electrical events is accomplished by structures within the Organ of Corti. The Organ of Corti sits atop the basilar membrane and runs the length of the cochlea. It is composed of the inner and outer hair cells which are specialized sensory receptor cells; the tectorial membrane which overlies the hair cells; and supporting structures that maintain the hair cells, the tectorial membrane, and the basilar membrane in optimal orientation.

The hair cells are actually mechanoreceptors sensitive to movement within the Organ of Corti. They receive their name from the rows of small hairs or cilia that protrude from the tops of the cells. The tallest cilia of the outer hair cells are embedded in the overlying tectorial membrane. All inner hair cell cilia, and the shorter outer hair cell cilia, are free-standing in the fluid space between the top of the hair cells and the tectorial membrane.

Movement of the basilar membrane alternately pulls down and pushes up the hair cells in response to inward and outward stapes motion. The tectorial membrane is anchored on one side to immobile bone and on the other side to the basilar membrane via supporting cells. It slides diagonally across the hair cells during basilar membrane motion. Since the tips of the tallest outer hair cell cilia are embedded in the tectorial membrane, movement of the basilar membrane and the consequent sliding of the tectorial membrane causes a shearing of the cilia. The free-standing cilia of the inner hair cells are also sheared but, in this case, by local fluid movement accompanying movement of Organ of Corti structures.

Ciliary movement directly affects the electrical characteristics of the hair cells. The mechanism by which this is accomplished is not entirely understood. It is likely that the shearing of the cilia distorts the top of the hair cell by pulling on it; this alters the flow of ions into the cell. The change in ion flow produces an electrical change in the hair cell called the receptor potential. Since the receptor potential is directly linked to ciliary movement (consequent to basilar membrane motion), it is approximately an analog representation of the basilar membrane movement directly below the hair cell. A sinusoidal sound, at frequencies below 5 kHz, producing sinusoidal basilar membrane motion will lead, therefore, to a sinusoidal receptor potential whose frequency, duration, and amplitude will correspond to the activating stimulus.

At the base of each hair cell are synapses formed by the dendrites of afferent nerve cells. The afferent nerve cells have their cell bodies in the spiral ganglion in the core or modiolus of the cochlea. Their axons leave the cochlea forming the auditory nerve, and project to the cochlear nucleus in the medulla. All auditory information transduced at the receptors is carried to the brain through these afferent auditory nerve cells.

The receptor potential causes the release of a chemical transmitter stored presynaptically in the hair cell. The transmitter crosses the synaptic cleft, a narrow fluid-filled space, and attaches to the afferent dendrite. The effect of the transmitter is to briefly alter the ionic flow into the dendrite, thereby producing a temporary electrical change in it. This electrical change, the generator potential, initiates all-or-none action potentials in the nerve cell. The release of the transmitter by the hair cells occurs during a restricted phase of the receptor potential that corresponds to unidirectional basilar membrane movement. The quantity of transmitter released is directly related to the receptor potential amplitude. So the temporal and amplitude characteristics of the generator potentials in the auditory nerve cell dendrites are systematically related to basilar membrane movement in one direction.

The dendrites of the auditory nerve cells enter the Organ of Corti through the habenula perforata, small openings in the cochlear bone adjacent to the inner hair cells. About 20 afferent dendrites pass through each of these openings. Almost all are radial fibers that proceed to the nearest inner hair cell where they form large synapses covering the lower two-thirds of the hair cell. A few dendrites, the spiral fibers, cross the Organ of Corti, travel basally about 100 hair cells, and then successively synapse upon the first, second, and third rows of outer hair cells. The synapses formed on the outer hair cells are quite small and are restricted to the base of the hair cell.[4]

The innervation ratios of the inner and the outer hair cells are quite different. Each inner hair cell receives synaptic contact from about 20 afferent fibers. The outer hair cells are innervated only by 3 or 4 afferents. Likewise, the radial and spiral fibers innervate different numbers and configurations of hair cells. Each radial fiber innervates and appears to be activated by only a single inner hair cell. Each spiral fiber appears to be activated by about 10 outer hair cells extending along a distance of 1 mm of the cochlea.

While independent innervation of inner and outer hair cells in the cochlea is apparent, studies of the response characteristics of auditory nerve cells have failed to reveal two functionally distinct cell populations corresponding to the radial and the spiral fibers. Instead, all auditory nerve cells appear to be influenced by both inner and outer hair cells. The search for an anatomic mechanism to account for the combination of inner and outer hair cell activity so far has been unsuccessful. There is no evidence of synaptic contact between radial and spiral fibers. The most likely explanation is that a direct electrical interaction between the hair cells themselves occurs, and this accounts for the observed functional interaction in the auditory nerve.[5]

ELECTRICAL ACTIVITY OF THE AUDITORY NERVE

The central component of the auditory system begins with the auditory nerve. Here, information about environmental sounds derived from basilar membrane motion is transduced into neural codes appropriate for processing in the central nervous system. Information transmitted to and within the central nervous system occurs in the form of very brief traveling electrical impulses called action potentials. Action potentials are always identical and are all-or-none, that is, they either occur or they do not occur. Their response to stimuli varies only in rate and temporal pattern. The rate and temporal pattern of the action potentials, and the nerve cells (neurons) in which they occur, constitute the information used by the brain to detect, locate, and identify environmental sounds.

Considerable research has been done to establish correlations between acoustic stimuli, neural responses, and auditory perception. These correlations have helped to define the specific neural codes and neural processing mechanisms of the auditory brain.

Studies of the action potential responses of single cells have utilized a microelectrode recording technique. In this technique, an extremely fine electrode is inserted into or adjacent to an individual neuron. Then the changes in electrical activity occurring in that cell in response to sounds are monitored and subjected to a variety of analytic procedures. Several analytical procedures are used to evaluate the relationship between auditory stimuli and subsequent action potential responses in an individual nerve cell. These procedures include: (1) the determination of the stimuli that generate activity in a specific cell; (2) the measurement of the amount of activity produced; and (3) the evaluation of the temporal pattern of the activity. Underlying each analytical procedure is the assumption that the response parameter that is measured is a functional neural code.

The sounds that activate a cell comprise the cell's response area. The boundaries of the response area are established by determining the minimum intensity, as a function of frequency, that is necessary to activate the cell. Each cell exhibits a "best" or "characteristic frequency": the stimulus frequency to which the cell responds at the lowest intensity and, therefore, the frequency to which it is most sensitive. The best frequency of each cell differs since each cell's dendrites innervate unique cochlear regions. However, the shapes of the response areas are basically similar. As the stimulus intensity is increased, a progressively broader range of frequencies, primarily those lower than the best frequency, activate the cell. This effect is also observed on the basilar membrane. The boundaries of the response area of an auditory nerve cell, however, do not correspond in a one-to-one manner to the frequency range activating a specific place on the basilar membrane. Rather, the neural response area reflects additional processing probably within the Organ of Corti which serves to restrict, particularly at low intensities, the range of frequencies to which the cell responds.

The restriction in the response area of auditory nerve fibers improves the auditory system's ability to code stimulus characteristics using a "place" mechanism. "Place coding" means that activity in a specific cell or group of cells (a specific place in the nervous system) signals to the brain the presence of a certain sound. The more restricted the range of stimuli to which a cell responds, the more precise the system's ability to code by place.

The restriction in response area that occurs between the basilar membrane and the auditory nerve, reflects the contribution of the outer hair cells to the auditory nerve cell response. Destruction of the outer hair cells results in a loss of the responsiveness of auditory nerve cells to low, but not high, intensity sounds.[6] This results in the decreased hearing sensitivity associated with a mild to moderate sensorineural hearing loss. In addition to a threshold shift, the absence of contributions from the more sharply tuned outer hair cells may decrease the individual's frequency resolving capacity. However, it is likely that some inner hair cell damage must also be sustained before frequency resolution is greatly affected.

The response of individual cells to a broad rather than narrow frequency range at suprathreshold sound intensities may be adaptively important. First, it protects the organism from total loss of hearing at certain frequencies if minor damage occurs to restricted cochlear or auditory nerve regions. Suprathreshold sounds are within the response areas of many nerve cells. Second, it provides a means of place coding in which the number of active cells signals sound intensity, while the array of active cells signals the frequency of the sound.

Both the temporal patterns of neural firing and the place of firings are affected by the frequency and intensity characteristics of the sound stimulus. For sounds below 5 kHz, the temporal features of basilar membrane movement are encoded in the temporal features of the elicited train of action potentials. Action potentials are initiated only during a restricted phase of basilar membrane motion.[7] So each action potential is synchronized with or locked into the stimulus features. When the stimulus is sinusoidal (a pure tone), the action potentials occur at temporal intervals either equal to the period of the sinusoid (the interval between cycles) or, since action potentials are rarely elicited by each stimulus cycle, at intervals equal to integral multiples of the stimulus period.

Phase locking in response to stimulus frequencies below 5kHz is observed in all auditory nerve neurons. At higher frequencies, phase locking does not occur because of the inherent limitations in the system's ability to isolate extremely rapid basilar membrane events. However, other temporal features of the sound, referred to as amplitude envelope characteristics, are encoded in the temporal discharge pattern. For example, the beginning and the end of a sound are revealed in the onset and the termination of the train of stimulus elicited action potentials. More detailed coding of amplitude envelope characteristics also probably occurs in the auditory nerve cells, but has been studied only in cells of the cochlear nucleus.

BRAIN STEM AUDITORY MECHANISMS

The cochlear nucleus is the region of the medulla to which all auditory nerve cell axons project and in which they terminate. It is the site of the initial interaction and integration of information carried separately by auditory nerve fibers. The cochlear nucleus contains three anatomically and probably functionally distinct regions: the anteroventral, the posteroventral, and the dorsal nuclei. Each auditory nerve axon branches and terminates upon cells in all three nuclear regions. These multiple projections result in a wide divergence of information from the auditory nerve to a variety of cochlear nucleus neurons. So most cochlear nucleus cells are influenced by many auditory nerve cells from which they receive converging inputs.

The integration or processing of information in cochlear nucleus neurons takes place in the cell body. Action potentials occurring presynaptically release a chemical transmitter that triggers a flow of ions into the cell. This produces a temporary electrical change in the cell membrane. The electrical change may be either a depolarization, an excitatory postsynaptic potential (EPSP), or a hyperpolarization, an inhibitory postsynaptic potential (IPSP). When the sum of the postsynaptic potentials, EPSPs and IPSPs, exceeds a threshold at some instant in time, an action potential is generated and transmitted down the axon. If the sum of the EPSPs and IPSPs fails to exceed a threshold, no action potential occurs. The occurrence of an action potential, therefore, depends on the summation of excitatory inputs from several sources, and may be blocked by simultaneous inhibitory inputs from other sources. The timing of the input to the neuron, then, is critical to processing since certain configurations of arriving inputs will cause the neurons to respond, while other input configurations will block a response.

The elaborate input arrays of many cochlear nucleus neurons makes possible the extraction of critical stimulus features from the neural activity transmitted by the auditory nerve. For example, many cochlear nucleus neurons preferentially respond to rapid frequency and intensity changes. These rapidly varying acoustic features are major components of speech and other adaptively significant sounds. Other cochlear nucleus neurons respond to continuous sounds and, like auditory nerve neurons, exhibit phase locking. There are then, within the cochlear nucleus, separate groups of neurons responsive to critical transient and sustained features of environmental sounds.[8]

The ability of cochlear nucleus neurons to exhibit in their response the temporal features of a sound, demonstrates an initial sound analysis. However, the importance of temporal resolution in the response is not *per se* to generate a neural code corresponding to acoustic features. Rather, it is to establish a pattern of neural firing that makes possible the distribution of stimulus information through appropriate neural channels via the postsynaptic integration process. The precise timing of excitatory and inhibitory inputs to each cell along the auditory pathway is critical if each cell is to respond when and only when the appropriate sound is present in the environment.

A well-studied example of the role of temporal interaction is the extraction of sound location from interaural time cues. Normally, an external sound reaches both ears. However, sound travels at a finite speed and, if it originates to the left of the head, it will reach the left ear up to 1 msec before it reaches the right ear. If it comes from a source at midline, it will reach both ears simultaneously. If it originates to the right, it will reach the right ear before reaching the left. The exact interaural time difference for sounds coming from off midline is dependent upon the location of the sound source on the horizontal plane and the interaural distance. Humans are able to discriminate interaural time differences as small as 20 μsec. This incredible temporal resolution ability is possible because of neural interactions that take place primarily in the medial superior olivary nucleus (MSO), an aggregate of cells located bilaterally in the medulla.

The neural mechanism responsible for extracting interaural time differences is similar to the delay-line model proposed more than 30 years ago.[9] Each MSO cell receives input from the anteroventral cochlear nuclei of both sides. The inputs from both sides exhibit similar temporal discharge patterns. When the discharges from both ears arrive at the MSO neuron simultaneously, summation occurs, and the medullary neuron responds by sending impulses to higher centers. When the discharges do not arrive simultaneously, summation fails to occur, and the binaural neuron does not respond. If the conduction time from each ear to the binaural neuron is exactly the same, the neuron will respond only when the sound arrives at both ears simultaneously, that is, when the sound source is directly in front. If it takes longer for the input from the right ear to reach the binaural neuron, then the binaural neuron will respond only when the sound is located to the right. The added conduction time compensates for the earlier arrival of the sound waves at the right ear.[10]

The delay-line mechanism results in the activation of specific MSO cells in accordance with the location in external space of the sound source. Obviously, this mechanism depends on the precise timing of bilateral neural inputs arriving at each MSO cell. Such precise timing is present in phase-locked firing to pure tones, and in time-locked firing to envelope and rapidly changing sound features. The delay-line mechanism, however, yields information that is ambiguous to some extent. For example, a sound coming directly from the front, directly from behind, or directly from above the head arrives at both ears simultaneously leading to the activation of the same MSO cells. In fact, front, top, and back discriminations are quite difficult. Accurate localization usually requires head movements, visual input, learning, or some combination of these factors. The need for information in addition to interaural time difference to resolve the ambiguity is noted in infants. Young infants are capable of making side to side localization discrimination, presumably utilizing their wired-in delay-line mechanisms. But front/back discriminations do not occur until somewhat later in development, and seem to require multisensory experience.

The localization of a sound source may also be accomplished by the analysis of interaural intensity differences. When a sound source is off to one side, an interaural intensity difference results from an "acoustic shadow" cast by the head. This shadow effect decreases the intensity of sounds arriving at the ear opposite the sound source. However, the acoustic shadow is substantial only for high-frequency sounds.

The analysis of interaural intensity differences takes place primarily in the lateral superior olive (LSO) of the superior olivary complex. The LSO, like the MSO, receives input from the anteroventral cochlear nucleus on both sides of the head. However, the contralateral input arrives at the LSO following a synaptic interruption at the medial nucleus of the trapezoid body (MNTB). The ipsilateral input to binaural LSO cells is always excitatory, while the contralateral input is always inhibitory. This suggests that a function of the MNTB is to convert the excitatory output of the anteroventral cochlear nucleus into an inhibitory form for relaying to the LSO. The presence of an excitatory ipsilateral input and an inhibitory contralateral input to each LSO cell means that a sound coming from the right will result in greater excitatory (compared to inhibitory) input to right LSO cells. A sound coming from the left provides a greater inhibitory input to right LSO cells. The reverse situation prevails at the left LSO. Presumably, the relative magnitudes of excitation and inhibition, and the resultant effect on neuron firing rate, signal the spatial location of the sound to higher levels of the brain.

The binaural mechanisms that distribute activity across different neurons as a function of sound source location are important not only in sound localization, but also in improving the detectability of consequential sounds in the presence of other competing sounds. Simultaneously occurring sounds emanating from different locations in space will activate different groups of cells. Higher mechanisms of attention then, may select the external sound of greatest importance from the array of active cells. Individuals with monaural hearing losses, or substantial differences in hearing ability between the two ears, are unable to use this mechanism. These individuals have significant problems when discriminating sounds in a noisy environment.

The outputs of the MSO and LSO ascend in the lateral lemniscus and terminate primarily in the inferior colliculus located bilaterally in the midbrain. In addition to superior olivary fibers, each inferior colliculus receives a direct monaural input from the contralateral dorsal cochlear nucleus. Superior olivary complex fibers arriving at the inferior colliculus bring information concerning the spatial location of the sound source. The role of the evolutionarily recent, rapid conducting, dorsal cochlear nucleus fibers is unclear. In lower vertebrates, the homologue of the inferior colliculus is the highest auditory processing center. Even in mammals, the inferior colliculus has major outputs to centers controlling acoustically triggered reflex motor acts, in addition to its role in refining auditory information for transmission to higher centers.

Nearly all inferior colliculus neurons are sensitive to the location in space of the sound source. Most of these cells in the right inferior colliculus are sensitive to sounds to the left of the organism, while in the left inferior colliculus, most cells are sensitive to sounds coming from the right.[11, 12] The role of the inferior colliculus in processing sounds originating in the contralateral spatial field, and in generating appropriate motor activity, can be observed by artificially stimulating the inferior colliculus with implanted electrodes. Electrical stimulation of one inferior colliculus initiates orienting reflexes including conjugate (parallel) eye movements, ear movements, and turning in the direction contralateral to the stimulated inferior colliculus.[13] This suggests that, under normal circumstances, sounds activate the inferior colliculus contralateral to the direction of the sound source and that activation of collicular neurons, in turn, elicits orienting behaviors in the direction of the sound.

Some of the motor output of the inferior colliculus is mediated through the deep layers of the superior colliculus and adjacent neural regions. Many of the cells in these areas are multimodal, receiving input from visual, tactile, and auditory centers. The input to multimodal cells is such that these cells respond to stimuli coming from the same location in space regardless of the modality that activates them. So some neurons respond to a sound, or to a visual display, or touch originating in a specific spatial location.[14, 15] Activation of these cells presumably leads to orienting movements in the direction of the stimulus.

EFFECTS OF DEVELOPMENT AND SENSORY DEPRIVATION

From the previous discussion, based primarily on research in adult organisms, it appears that localization abilities and consequent orienting responses are wired in to the nervous system. However, wired-in mechanisms are inherently inflexible and, therefore, potentially unadaptive. This is particularly true in the developing organism. For example, during growth the interaural distance gradually increases. A neural mechanism that from birth signals to the brain that each interaural time difference means a sound is coming from a specific location would be inaccurate. Furthermore, the eventual interaural distance at maturity is not known at birth because the genes controlling the establishment of the brain stem neural mechanisms are not coordinated with, nor can they influence, the genes controlling mature head size and shape. Fortunately, the binaural neural mechanisms are modifiable during development by environmental stimuli. This plasticity allows the developing organism to compensate neurally for physical changes occurring during growth.

Neural plasticity during development has been studied most extensively in the binocular visual system. The binocular visual system presents a problem analogous to the binaural auditory system. It must compensate neurally for developmental changes in the interocular distance and for minor deviations between the eyes. The binocular system compensates for growth and for slight interocular deviations by altering the input to each cell so that retinal regions receiving images from similar portions of the visual field project to the same cells. However, when the deviation between the eyes is too great, or if one eye has been covered to prevent binocular reception, input from the deviant eye is shut off. This central mechanism prevents the transmission of irreconcilable visual images. Neural plasticity occurs only during a critical developmental period; after that period the capacity for compensatory neural change no longer exists.[16, 17]

Similar effects also seem to occur in the auditory system.[18] Occluding one ear canal to prevent the normal binaural reception of sounds during the critical developmental period prevents the establishment of normal binaural connections, and reduces the number of binaurally sensitive cells present when the occluded ear is opened. Blocking of an ear canal after the critical period, or blocking of both ear canals, has no effect on binaural sensitivity. Normally, almost all inferior colliculus cells are binaurally sensitive and exhibit temporal discharge patterns highly sensitive to binaural stimulus parameters. One might speculate that some other auditory abilities, in addition to sound localization, might be affected by the absence of normal binaural input during the critical period. The early assessment and treatment of disorders affecting auditory input, therefore, seems critical to ensure normal development of brain stem neural mechanisms.

The infant with an intact binaural system also has an advantage in acquiring knowledge about the environment. The ability to orient to sounds, and thereby bring into register both auditory and visual information, facilitates some aspects of early cognitive development. Furthermore, the ability to use binaural mechanisms to separate simultaneous sounds coming from different spatial locations is important in establishing the relationship between sounds and the objects that produce them. A normal binaural system is also important to mechanisms of attention that allow one to focus on certain sounds while ignoring others.

In addition to the developmental plasticity of the binaural localization mechanism, there is some evidence that the sensitivity to specific sounds found among neurons in the inferior colliculus is influenced by the presence of these sounds in the environment during early development.[19] Animals exposed to specific sounds during a critical period tend, as adults, to have an unusually large proportion of cells responsive to these sounds. In the visual system, distorted input during development caused by lens deformation produces permanent changes in the visual system and in visual perception. These changes are unaffected by correction of the lens after the critical period.[20] One might anticipate permanent auditory system and auditory perceptual changes as a result of abnormal auditory input caused by early middle or inner ear pathology. These neurally-based changes may persist even after treatment of the disorder, or compensation for the deficit through amplification after the critical period.

The functioning of cells in the inferior colliculus is affected not only by abnormal sensory input, but also by perinatal oxygen deficits.[21] Marked and progressive degeneration of inferior colliculus cells has been observed in monkeys following recovery from perinatal asphyxia. The period of asphyxiation that produced degeneration in the inferior colliculus was substantially less than the amount of deprivation necessary to cause cellular degeneration in most other brain regions. These findings suggest that certain auditory structures are unusually sensitive to perinatal oxygen deficits, and that these deficits are likely to produce permanent changes in auditory functioning.

THALAMIC AND CORTICAL AUDITORY MECHANISMS

The outputs of the inferior colliculus to the superior colliculus have been described. However, the major inferior colliculus output projects to the thalamus, primarily the medial geniculate body. From the thalamus, the outputs ascend to auditory cortical regions in the temporal lobe. Little is known about the functioning of the medial geniculate body and other thalamic auditory centers. They do, however, have reciprocal connections with cells in the auditory cortex. This means that the auditory thalamus may be regarded as a functional component of the auditory cortical system rather than as a relay nucleus in the ascending auditory pathway.

Study of higher levels of the auditory pathway is complicated by the fact that most cells respond poorly in anesthetized preparations. Even in awake, behaving organisms, single cell responses may be poor unless the stimulus is of significance to the animal under study. For example, cells may be more responsive to a sound if the animal has been trained to expect a certain consequence or to perform a certain behavior upon hearing the sound.[22] This demonstrates the influence of higher brain processes, including attention, memory, and learning, on the activity of cells of the auditory cortex.

Because of the difficulties in assessing the role of the auditory cortex through the analysis of single cell activity, most knowledge of auditory cortical functioning has been obtained through evaluation of behavioral changes observed in animals following destruction of specified auditory cortical regions. Obviously, such animal studies yield no information concerning the neural mechanisms underlying speech discrimination or language processing, but they do show that temporal pattern discrimination—but not frequency, intensity, or localization discriminations—are impaired by cortical lesions.[23] Animals with auditory cortex lesions are unable to correctly respond to variations in stimulus sequence, but are able to discriminate between pairs of sounds differing in frequency, intensity, or spatial location. However, impairments in some simple discrimination tasks are observed if, in addition to the discrimination, complex motor acts are required such as walking to the correct place upon hearing a certain sound. Auditory discriminiation abilities have in many studies been confounded with the ability to learn or carry out certain motor acts in response to sounds. The auditory cortex unquestionably plays a significant role in the acquisition and retention of sound-initiated motor responses that are more complex than simple orienting responses.

THE EFFERENT SYSTEM

In the preceding discussions, emphasis was placed on the role of the ascending auditory pathway in processing sounds. Paralleling the ascending pathways are descending or efferent pathways that carry information from higher auditory centers to successively lower brain regions. These pathways apparently modify or regulate neural activity at each auditory level, including the peripheral receptors.

The anatomic substrates of the afferent auditory system are well-documented, but the role of the efferent system in audition is unknown. The best understood component of this pathway is the olivocochlear system. This system transmits activity from the superior olivary complex to the hair cells and the bipolar cell dendrites of the cochlea. The primary effect of olivocochlear activation is the inhibition of receptor activity in the outer hair cells. Since the outer hair cells transduce low-intensity sounds, olivocochlear system activation presumably decreases auditory sensitivity to such stimuli. The greatest influence of the olivocochlear system is on outer hair cells located in the basal or high frequency cochlear region. This suggests that the olivocochlear system plays a role in decreasing sensitivity to extraneous high-frequency sounds, possibly improving auditory discrimination in the presence of high-frequency noise.

CONCLUSIONS

This chapter has reviewed current knowledge of the neuroanatomic and neurophysiologic mechanisms that comprise the auditory input system. It has described the conversion of sound waves into electrical activity, and the coding in this activity for some critical sound features. What has been described, however, is only one component of the raw material upon which higher association areas of the brain operate to produce the individually unique conscious sensations called hearing. Other factors—including memory, arousal, attention, emotional state, other sensory activity, and cognition—also contribute to hearing. Through knowledge of the input system, one can establish how it influences hearing, and how disruptions in this system may affect hearing, but one can never thoroughly understand or describe hearing as a function of the input mechanism alone.

REFERENCES

1. Starr A: Regulatory mechanisms of the auditory pathway, in Locke S (ed): Modern Neurology. Boston, Little, Brown, 1969, p 101
2. Borg E, Zakrisson JE: The stapedius muscle and speech perception, in Bench RJ, Pye A, Pye JD (eds): Sound Reception in Mammals. New York, Academic Press, 1975, p51
3. von Békésy G: Experiments in Hearing. New York, McGraw-Hill, 1960
4. Spoendlin H: Neuroanatomical basis of cochlear coding mechanisms. Audiology 14:383–407, 1975
5. Sellick PM, Russell IJ: Intracellular studies of cochlear hair cells: Filling the gap between basilar membrane mechanics and neural excitation, in Naunton RF, Fernandez C (eds): Evoked Electrical Activity in the Auditory Nervous System. New York, Academic Press, 1978, p113
6. Dallas P, Harris D: Properties of auditory nerve responses in absence of outer hair cells. J Neurophysiol 41:365–383, 1978
7. Rose JE, Brugge JF, Anderson DJ, et al: Phase-locked responses to low-frequency tones in single auditory nerve fibers of the squirrel monkey. J Neurophysiol 30:769–793, 1967

8. Møller AR: Coding of time-varying sounds in the cochlear nucleus. Audiology 17:446–468, 1977
9. Jeffress LA: A place theory of sound localization. J Comp Physiol Psychol 41:35–39, 1948
10. Goldberg JM, Brown PB: Responses of binaural neurons of dog superior olivary complex to dichotic tonal stimuli: Some physiological mechanisms of sound localization. J Neurophysiol 32:613–636, 1969
11. Stillman RD: Characteristic delay neurons in the inferior colliculus of the kangaroo rat. Exp Neurol 32:404–412, 1971
12. Stillman RD: Responses of high-frequency inferior colliculus neurons to interaural intensity differences. Exp Neurol 36:118–126, 1972
13. Syka J, Straschill M: Activation of superior colliculus neurons and motor responses after electrical stimulation of the inferior colliculus. Exp Neurol 29:384–392, 1970
14. Gordon B: Receptive fields in deep layers of cat superior colliculus. J Neurophysiol 36:157–178, 1973
15. Dräger UC, Hubel DH: Responses to visual stimulation and relationship between visual, auditory, and somatosensory inputs in mouse superior colliculus. J Neurophysiol 38:690–713, 1975
16. Hubel DH, Wiesel TN: The period of susceptibility to the physiological effects of unilateral eye closure in kittens. J Physiol 206:419–436, 1970
17. Banks MS, Aslin RN: Sensitive period for the development of human binocular vision. Science 190:675–677, 1975
18. Clopton BM, Silverman MS: Plasticity of binaural interaction. II. Critical period and changes in midline response. J Neurophysiol 40:1275–1280, 1977
19. Clopton BM, Winfield JA: Effect of early exposure to patterned sound on unit activity in rat inferior colliculus. J Neurophysiol 39:1081–1089, 1976
20. Freeman RD, Mitchell DE, Millodot M: A neural effect of partial visual deprivation in humans. Science 175:1384–1386, 1972
21. Sechzer JA, Ford MD, Windle WF: Studies of monkeys asphyxiated at birth: Implications for minimal cerebral dysfunction, in Walzer S, Wolff PH (eds): Minimal Cerebral Dysfunction in Children. New York, Grune and Stratton, 1973, p19
22. Miller JM, Sutton D, Pfingst B, et al: Single cell activity in the auditory cortex of rhesus monkeys: Behavioral dependency. Science 177:449–451, 1972
23. Neff WD: The brain and hearing: Auditory discriminations affected by brain lesions. Ann Otol Rhinol Laryngol 86:500–506, 1977

Robert Stillman

2
Auditory Evoked Potentials

Sounds evoke orderly sequences of electrochemical events in the brain that begin at the cochlear receptors and continue through the brain stem and the cortical auditory regions. These electrochemical events—including receptor potentials, action potentials, postsynaptic potentials, and dendritic field potentials—underlie the reception, transmission, and processing of sounds. Recently, remotely recorded signs of this electrochemical activity, the auditory evoked potentials (AEP), have been utilized both to further our understanding of auditory system functioning and to provide a unique tool for the assessment of human auditory disorders.

Remote recordings of the electrical activity of the brain have been obtained for many years. This activity, recorded from electrodes attached to the surface of the head, is called the electroencephalogram or EEG. It is the sum of all electrical activity occurring in the brain at each instant in time. Included in the EEG is activity generated by the sensory and motor systems, and by the numerous endogenous cortical processes which underlie the complex operations of the brain. Neural activity in response to sounds, the AEP, is embedded in the EEG. It may be extracted, however, by suitable recording, amplifying, and computer averaging procedures.

The AEP is a series of waves coinciding temporally with neural activity in peripheral, brain stem, and cortical auditory regions. Each wave reflects the collective activity of a large number of cells responding in unison to sounds. Three groups of AEP waves have been identified and categorized

---

Preparation of this chapter was supported, in part, by NINCDS Grant 1R01 NS15681-01

according to the time interval or latency between sound onset and the appearance of the AEP wave. The earliest waves are the brain stem evoked potentials (BEP). They occur within 10 msec following the onset of the sound, and reflect activation of peripheral and brain stem auditory structures. The second group of APEs are the middle latency evoked potentials (MLEP). They occur between 10 and 80 msec after sound onset, and are probably generated in thalamic and cortical auditory structures. The third group are the late evoked potentials. They begin at about 80 msec and continue until about 250 msec after the stimulus. The late evoked potentials reflect activity primarily in the association regions of the cerebral cortex. A fourth, even later group of waves, the event-related potentials (ERP), appear between about 280 and 1000 msec. The ERP, unlike the AEP, reflects psychologic processes underlying the analysis of sounds.

This chapter will describe the various evoked and event-related potentials initiated by sounds. Emphasis will be placed on identifying the neural sources, the functional significance, the developmental course and the clinical application of these potentials. Literally thousands of papers on evoked potentials have been published in the past 20 years. Only a small proportion of them can be reviewed here. Electrocochleography, sonomotor potentials, and much of the older work on late evoked potentials will receive only brief mention. The wealth of literature on evoked potentials initiated by activation of the visual and somesthetic systems are also excluded from this review. The reader is encouraged to consult the bibliography and references cited at the end of the chapter for both supplemental and in-depth information on evoked potentials.

RECORDING TECHNIQUES

Recording evoked potentials is technically quite simple and causes no discomfort to the subject. EEG disk electrodes are affixed to the scalp at conventional locations. In general, the active electrode is placed at vertex: designated as the intersection on the scalp of two lines, one drawn between the ear canals and the other between the bridge of the nose and the inion. Reference electrodes are usually placed on the mastoid or on the ear lobes. Other electrode configurations are also used to extract specific AEP components.

The minute electrical activity recorded by the electrodes is differentially amplified, usually 100,000 times, and computer averaged over 20 to 4000 successive stimulus presentations. Computer averaging helps to resolve the AEP by removing from the response the electrical activity that is not synchronized to the stimulus. Averaging, however, limits the recoverable neural events to those that remain highly synchronized to the repeated stimuli and do not habituate rapidly when the same sound is presented repeatedly.

Simple acoustic stimuli are typically employed to elicit the AEP. These stimuli are of two types: transient and sustained. Transient stimuli are brief clicks generated by a square wave pulse or short (1 to 4 msec) tone burst. Transient stimuli have very broad spectral characteristics and activate extensive regions of the basilar membrane. Sustained stimuli generally are pure tones of 20 to 200 msec duration. Their spectral characteristics are narrow and, except at high intensities, activate restricted basilar membrane regions. A few studies have used complex stimuli including speech sounds.

BRAIN STEM EVOKED POTENTIALS

The full complement of brain stem evoked potentials was first described by Jewett and Williston.[1] The waveforms they observed exhibited seven peaks designated sequentially, waves I to VII. The waves begin less than 2 msec following an acoustic click and are complete within 10 to 12 msec. Wave V is the most prominent of the waves and is observed within 5 to 10 dB of perceptual threshold. BEPs are recorded in all audiologically and neurologically normal subjects, but in some subjects, waves IV and V are fused, while in others, waves VI and/or VII are indistinct. Within subjects, the waveform characteristics are essentially invariant from session to session.

The latency of each BEP wave (the time between the onset of the sound and the appearance of the wave) decreases in a systematic manner with intensity increments. Furthermore, the absolute latency values at each stimulus intensity are essentially invariant across subjects. It is this remarkable intersubject response stability that has permitted the establishment of latency-intensity norms for each BEP wave, and the use of deviations from the norm as a sensitive indicator of auditory system pathology.

Clinical Application of the BEP

Evoked potential evaluation of peripheral and brain stem auditory functioning is an objective procedure in the sense that active participation or cooperation of the subject is not required. Evoked potential techniques, therefore, have important applications among individuals for whom the usual battery of behavioral audiometric tests yields uncertain results (for example, with neonates, infants, and multiply handicapped individuals). BEP results clearly distinguish between sensorineural, conductive, mixed, and retrocochlear pathology, and may be used to establish the presence or absence of recruitment. Subtle brain stem neurologic changes may also be uncovered by analysis of the BEP, often before the appearance of obvious behavioral symptoms.

The BEP, however, does not measure hearing. It is a probe which permits the identification of peripheral and brain stem pathology. Hearing is a complex psychologic phenomenon originating at higher brain levels. The extent to which the neural activity underlying the BEP contributes to hearing is unclear.

The BEP wave V latency and the interwave interval between waves I and V are the two BEP response parameters most useful in the clinical assessment of peripheral and brain stem auditory functioning. Other measures, including wave I to V amplitude ratios and stimulus rate effects on amplitude and latency, yield additional information particularly relevant to the evaluation of the neurologic integrity of the brain stem.

Knowledge of the factors that determine the latency of the waves is necessary in order to understand the rationale for clinical applications of BEP latency measures. Two factors contribute to the BEP wave latencies: neural conduction time and basilar membrane travel time. Neural conduction time is the time required for neural impulses to travel between each BEP wave generator. It determines the temporal interval between successive BEP waves. Neural conduction time is a function of axon characteristics (length, diameter, and degree of myelination), and the number and physiologic characteristics of the interposed synapses. Basilar membrane travel time is the time difference between the arrival of the sound-initiated mechanical motion at the cochlea, and the generation of neural activity. Mechanical characteristics of the basilar membrane dictate that the basal, high-frequency cochlear regions are activated as much as 4 msec before the apical, low-frequency regions.

Neural conduction time and basilar membrane travel time may be separately analyzed and applied to the identification of specific auditory system impairments. Neural conduction time, usually measured by the temporal interval between waves I and V, is constant regardless of the frequency or intensity of the stimulus.[2] Abnormally long interwave intervals are associated with pathologic processes affecting the speed of impulse conduction, and are observed in patients with demyelinating diseases such as multiple sclerosis.[3] Abnormally long interwave intervals are also observed in individuals with specific or diffuse neurologic disorders of congenital, perinatal, or postnatal origin. Abnormally short interwave intervals have been associated with Down's syndrome.[4] There is as yet no neurologic explanation for these findings.

When the interwave intervals are normal, the latency of the prominent wave V provides an accurate measure of the basilar membrane regions contributing to the observed evoked potential. In audiologically normal subjects, wave V is initiated primarily by activity in the basilar membrane regions most sensitive to stimuli of 2 to 8 kHz.[5] When high-frequency sensorineural pathology (affecting the integrity of the receptor cells or their neural connections) is present, the latency of wave V is abnormally long. The prolonged latency means that the basilar membrane region initiating the BEP is more apical than normal due to a functional impairment in basally located structures. Wave V latency, therefore, provides an estimate of the region and extent of sensorineural pathology. The slope of wave V latency-intensity functions may be used to establish recruitment as well as to indicate the presence of conductive impairments.[6, 7]

Development of the BEP

The BEP first appears at about 26 weeks gestational age. However, at this time, both wave V latencies and the interwave intervals are somewhat greater than for adults. The BEP latencies and interwave intervals decrease with age and achieve normal adult values at 18 to 24 months.[8]

The prolonged BEP latencies in the developing infant reflect, in part, initiation of the response by more apical cochlear regions. This may be due to inefficient transmission to the cochlea of high-frequency sounds, or incomplete basal cochlear development. Slower neural conduction time in young infants also contributes to the prolonged latencies.[9]

Developmental differences in BEP wave latencies and interwave intervals have led to the establishment of age-specific latency-intensity norms.[10] This has made it possible to detect peripheral and brain stem auditory disorders almost at birth, and to monitor the effect of therapy with potentially ototoxic drugs on auditory functioning in neonates and infants.

Neural Sources of the BEP

A variety of techniques have been employed to specify the brain stem origins of the BEP waves. These have included mapping of the BEP across the surface of the head,[11] identifying waveform abnormalities in humans with known brain stem lesions,[2, 12] and examining the BEP following controlled lesions in experimental animals.[13] The results of these studies have led to the unanimous conclusion that wave I is generated by auditory nerve activity. The generators of waves II to VII, however, are less easily defined. Waves II to VII probably reflect summed activity simultaneously occurring in several distinct brain stem regions. For example, wave II emanates primarily from the cochlear nucleus, although some late auditory nerve activity may be superimposed on it. While wave III originates bilaterally in the superior olivary complex, the superior olivary nuclei, which contribute to wave III are unclear. Waves IV and V probably reflect lateral lemniscus and inferior colliculus activity, but a contribution from the superior olivary complex cannot be ruled out. Waves VI and VII probably are generated in midbrain and/or thalamic auditory structures, but again the precise location is unclear.

FREQUENCY-FOLLOWING POTENTIALS (FFP)

The BEP waves represent the summed activity of high-frequency sensitive nerve cells responding in unison to the onset of transient sounds. A second type of brain stem evoked potential is elicited by sustained, low-frequency sounds. At low intensities, this potential is a plateau-like wave, equal in duration to the stimulus.[14, 15] It is present at 10 to 20 dB above threshold for normal hearing subjects and, at these intensities, reflects frequency-specific apical cochlear activity. At higher intensities, greater than 25 to 40 dB SL, a series of peaks occurring at temporal intervals equal to the period of the cycles of the tone is superimposed on the plateau-like response.[14] This potential is the frequency-following potential (FFP) and is observed in response to tones below about 1.5 kHz.

The FFP has not been widely used in auditory assessments. However, the FFP has several potentially important clinical applications. First, at low and moderate intensities, the FFP reflects brain stem neural responses derived from apical cochlear activity.[16, 17] Therefore, the FFP appears to be applicable to the assessment of cochlear regions inaccessible through use of the BEP. Second, the FFP reflects the response of a distinct subpopulation of auditory brain stem elements—neurons which respond in a phase-locked (frequency-following) manner for the duration of sustained sounds. Third, the FFP is unique among the AEPs in that it reveals, in detail, a brain stem level temporal neural code—phase-locking. This code is thought to be of consequence in pitch perception and sound localization. It has been suggested that abnormalities in the FFP or the absence of the FFP might be associated with auditory processing disorders.[15] Additional research is needed to establish what relationship, if any, the FFP has to normal and abnormal processing of sounds.

The FFP, like the BEP, is composed of activity generated in several brain stem neural regions.[18] However, because the eliciting stimulus is sustained, the activity evoked from separate generators overlaps in time. It is difficult, therefore, to clearly distinguish the contribution of each generator in the scalp-recorded response. Nonvertex scalp recordings and the evaluation of brain stem lesions in experimental animals are techniques that have been used to extract and localize the FFP sources.[18, 19] It appears that the FFP originates predominantly in lower brain stem regions including the cochlear nucleus and the superior olivary complex. There is, however, some contribution to the FFP at high intensities from the cochlear microphonic potential generated by receptor cells in the cochlea.

The FFP, like the BEP, has been recorded from human neonates,[20] and like the BEP, the neonatal FFP generally exhibits somewhat longer latencies than those observed in adults. Developmental changes in the FFP have not been explored systematically, nor has the FFP been used to assess neonatal and infant auditory system functioning.

In addition to sustained tones, other acoustic stimuli have been used to evoke activity originating in the apical regions of the cochlea. These stimuli include filtered clicks, brief tone pips, and broad-band clicks delivered in the presence of high-pass, band-pass, or notched masking noise. These stimuli evoke BEP-like responses, often with a succeeding FFP component. The latencies of these responses suggest that they are more frequency specific than the click evoked BEP. However, the clinical application of these responses awaits the establishment of norms on individuals with normal hearing and with known auditory system pathology.

MIDDLE LATENCY EVOKED POTENTIALS (MLEP)

The middle latency evoked potentials (MLEP) occur between 10 and 80 msec, and are composed of as many as eight successive positive and negative waves (N_o, P_o, N_a, N_b, P_b, N_c, P_c). The waveforms are similar in response to either transient or sustained sounds. The MLEP waves are unquestionably of neural origin. However, since sound-evoked reflexive contractions of the scalp musculature (sonomotor responses) also occur within the 10 to 80 msec time domain, precautions must be taken to prevent contamination of MLEP recordings by these sonomotor responses.

The MLEP wave generators have not yet been defined. The latencies of the potentials suggest origins in thalamocortical auditory regions. However, attempts to correlate MLEP waves with intracranial potentials recorded during human brain surgery have not been successful.[21] Studies of the MLEP in experimental animals with discrete brain lesions suggest that some contribution to the MLEP comes from the medial geniculate body and the primary auditory cortex contralateral to the stimulated ear.[22, 23]

Because of its high amplitude, stability and appearance at near behavioral audiometric threshold, the MLEP has shown some promise for frequency-specific assessment of peripheral auditory pathology. However, it now appears that the BEP provides the clinician with more precise and detailed information concerning cochlear integrity than does the MLEP. Possibly the MLEP will prove useful in evaluating auditory dysfunction originating in thalamic and cortical auditory regions.

The earlier MLEP components are clearly present in neonates and infants.[24, 25] In contrast to the BEP, the early MLEP waves exhibit shorter latencies in neonates and infants, than in adults.

LATE EVOKED POTENTIALS (LEP)

The late evoked potentials (LEP) were first identified more than 40 years ago,[26] and are the most thoroughly studied and widely applied of all evoked potentials. The LEP is composed of three relatively high amplitude waves: N_1, P_2, and N_2. These waves occur in response to auditory, visual, somesthetic, and vestibular stimulation. They have latencies between 80 and 250 msec and are best recorded at vertex. All three waves are evoked by both transient and sustained sounds. However, in response to sustained sounds, a negative wave equal in duration to the stimulus follows N_2.[27]

The LEP differs from the earlier BEP, FFP, and MLEP, in that its amplitude is influenced by psychologic factors as well as the acoustic characteristics of the stimulus. For example, the arousal and attention states of the subject have a distinct affect on the LEP, and the control of these factors is essential to the interpretation of LEP findings.

The LEP habituates in response to repeated presentations of the same stimulus. Therefore, the LEP, unlike the earlier potentials, may not always be obtained when there is activity in the auditory input system. The effects of habituation, arousal, and attention make the LEP less advantageous than the earlier potentials for audiometric testing. However, this does not preclude applications of the LEP in assessing higher level, complex auditory processes.

Habituation

The N_1-P_2 wave amplitude decreases dramatically when identical stimuli are presented at rates more rapid than one every ten seconds.[28] The amplitude decrement is almost 80 percent between rates of one per ten seconds and two per second; more rapid stimulus presentation rates may result in the total disappearance of the LEP. In contrast, the BEP, FFP, and MLEP are stable at rates above ten per second. Habituation of the N_1-P_2 response reflects the failure of contributing cortical neurons to respond to rapidly presented, unchanging stimuli. Acoustically different stimuli interposed between successive presentations of the original (test) stimulus also reduce the N_1-P_2 amplitude, but only when both stimuli activate overlapping pools of neurons. The effect is similar to increasing the stimulus presentation rate for identical stimuli.

The measurement of LEP habituation to test stimuli in the presence of intervening stimuli, has led to several interesting findings on cortical auditory processing. For example, two perceptually similar sounds, a 200 Hz tone and a 200 Hz burst of square-wave pulses filtered to confine spectral energy to the 1 kHz region, apparently activate essentially independent pools of cortical neurons. The intervening 200 Hz pulse burst does not substantially reduce the LEP amplitude to the 200 Hz test tone. In contrast, perceptually dissimilar sounds, the 200 Hz pulse burst and a 1 kHz tone do activate overlapping pools of neurons since the 1 kHz tone-evoked LEP is reduced by the intervening 200 Hz pulse burst.[29] These findings suggest that the perceptual similarity of two acoustically different stimuli is not the result of processing by common neural regions contributing to the LEP. Furthermore, it appears that acoustically similar but perceptually distinct sounds, may activate the same cortical neurons.

The habituation paradigm has also been used to demonstrate that multisensory association neurons contribute to the N_1-P_2 response.[30] For example, an intervening somesthetic stimulus affects the N_1-P_2 response to sounds, while an intervening visual stimulus has no effect on this auditory evoked response.

A more recent use of the habituation paradigm has been to derive the frequency response areas of LEP components.[31] In order to derive the response area, the frequency range of the intervening stimuli which affect the amplitude of the response to a test frequency is determined. Such studies have shown that the response areas of the N_1, the P_2 and the sustained LEP components differ in characteristic ways. This suggests that each component reflects activity in distinct, functionally different neural generators.

One obvious application of the habituation paradigm is in the analysis of speech sound processing, for example, to seek neural correlates of categorical perception. Such studies have not yet been attempted. However, the habituation paradigm might be used to determine if habituation to acoustically similar phonemes on opposite sides of a perceptual boundary is different from that obtained with acoustically similar phonemes that are less perceptually distinct (within boundaries). The results might be interpreted to indicate if phonetic coding occurs in the neural regions generating the LEP.

Effects of Arousal, Attention and Task

All LEP waves are affected by the subject's arousal level. The N_1 and P_2 waves are substantially greater in subjects who are awake and alert than in sleeping subjects. The amount of N_1 and P_2 amplitude decrement in sleep, relative to the awake state, is directly related to the depth of sleep.[27] The reverse is true for the N_2 wave which increases substantially during sleep becoming the most prominent LEP component. These findings suggest functional differences between the LEP components since they are differentially affected by arousal level.

Whether or not the subject is attending to or listening to the sound also affects the LEP amplitude. For example, if a subject is required to listen carefully to the sounds presented in order to perform some task, the N_1 and P_2 waves will be of greater amplitude than if the subject is instructed to ignore the sounds and concentrate on some other activity, such as reading. The N_2 wave is unaffected by the subject's attention to the stimulus.[32]

Many studies of the effect of attention on the N_1-P_2 response have been conducted. These studies have provided a basic understanding of the neural correlates of attention, and have been used to support various theories of attentional processes. Unfortunately, attention studies require trained, reliable listeners. Even under these conditions, intersubject variability is high. Thus, it is unlikely these studies can be applied where they are most needed: to determine if a patient with an intact auditory input system, but absent or inconsistent behavioral responses to sounds, fails to respond because of an attentional problem.

Neural Sources of the LEP

The neural generators of the LEP continue to be the subject of controversy. Mapping the LEP across the surface of the head indicates that the potentials are widely distributed across central and frontal scalp regions. The broad distribution of the LEP suggests that the waves are a composite of activity generated simultaneously in a number of cortical regions. These regions probably include primary auditory cortex, and temporal and frontal association areas.[27]

Development of the LEP

The LEP, like the BEP, decreases in latency with age.[33] These shifts are quite substantial: as much as 200 msec for N_2 between birth and 40 months of age. The age at which normal adult latency values are achieved has not been established, although it appears to occur by age six.[34]

The LEP in neonates is highly variable, and in the majority of neonates LEP waves cannot be distinguished even in response to moderately intense sounds.[35] This severely restricts the use of the LEP to evaluate neonates audiometrically, and to establish the funcitonal integrity of cortical auditory regions.

EVENT-RELATED POTENTIALS (ERP)

The event-related P_3 or P_{300} potential (ERP) is a unique among scalp-recorded neuroelectrical events. It appears only in response to perceptual decisions by the subject and, unlike brain stem and LEP waves, is unaffected by the physical characteristics of the stimulus.

The typical experimental procedure for eliciting an ERP is the oddball paradigm commonly employed in psychophysical detection experiments. Two discriminable stimuli are presented in sequence. One, the signal, is presented infrequently among the others, the nonsignals. The subject is instructed to count the number of times the signal is presented. The separate recording of the potentials evoked to signals and to nonsignals reveals a vertex positive wave in response to the signals, but not to the nonsignals. This wave follows N_2, and has a latency of about 300 msec. The late positive wave, the P_3 or P_{300} ERP, indicates the subject's detection of the signal among the nonsignals. The BEP and MLEP waves are essentially the same for signals and nonsignals.[32]

The ERP indicates perceptual decision processes and, unlike the LEP, is not a sensory evoked potential modulated by arousal and attentional states. An ERP can be elicited in the absence of sensory input if the signal is an omitted click in a train of clicks presented at equal intervals. In this case, ERP occurs as expected, about 300 msec following each omitted click, but is not preceded by brain stem or LEP waves.[32]

Not all ERPs require a conscious perceptual decision. An ERP is also observed in response to infrequent stimuli or unexpected changes in a repetitive stimulus sequence, even when the subject is instructed to ignore the stimuli. This ERP, the P_{3a}, differs from the ERP to counted signals, the P_3, in that it is of shorter latency and has a more frontal scalp distribution.[36] The P_{3a} may reflect some component of an alerting or orienting response to unpredictable or unexpected changes in ambient stimulation. The P_3 has a more central scalp distribution and appears to reflect a cognitive decision process.

Both the P_{3a} and P_3 may be applicable to the assessment of discrimination abilities. A P_3 is evoked when the subject is capable of discriminating between presented stimuli, even when the discrimination is difficult. However, the ability of the subject to cooperate in the task is required. The P_{3a} occurs in response to an unexpected stimulus change regardless of whether or not the subject is cooperating. However, in experiments conducted so far, only stimuli which differ from each other substantially have been used to elicit the P_{3a}.

The ERP has been used not only to demonstrate neural events associated with detection and discrimination, but also neural events related to recognition. The most comprehensive study utilized visual rather than auditory stimuli. However, similar ERP responses to sounds would be expected. In this study,[37] four types of stimuli were presented: (1) the number 2; (2) the number 4; (3) easily recognizable stimuli such as the word "THE", simple geometric figures, and line drawings; and (4) novel, unrecognizable quasi-random patterns. The subjects were instructed to count the 4s, which were presented infrequently, and to ignore the frequently presented 2s. The two other types of stimuli were occasionally presented between the 2s and 4s, but the subject was not warned to expect them. Separate analysis of potentials generated by each stimulus type revealed, as expected, an ERP with central scalp distribution in response to the 4s, and no ERP in response to the 2s. In response to the easily recognized words and figures, an ERP was also observed, but its scalp distribution was slightly more frontal. The ERP to novel unrecognizable stimuli had a substantially greater frontal distribution. However, when the same novel stimulus was interspersed repeatedly so that it was no longer novel or unrecognizable, the ERP elicited by it was more centrally distributed.

These results suggest that stimuli which are meaningful, either because of instructions to the subject (4s) or because they are familiar and easily recognized, elicit ERPs with predominantly central or parietal distributions. Stimuli which are unrecognizable and initially have no meaning activate more frontal cortical regions possibly associated with arousal. The shift in ERP scalp distribution, as a novel stimulus becomes familiar, may be associated with the establishment of meaning. Another interpretation of the shift in scalp distribution, however, is that the shift reflects changes in expectations about future stimulus events. Once the stimuli are expected and so are no longer novel, they need not be directed to frontal cortical regions concerned with arousal. The prospect of applying the ERP response to assess the meaningfulness of linguistic and nonlinguistic stimuli is exciting.

No studies have yet established with certainty that any ERP component reflects specific language mechanisms. Studies that have attempted to identify scalp-recorded events associated with linguistic processing tend to have many shortcomings. One major methodological problem is due to the necessity for response averaging to extract the ERP. Identical linguistic stimuli are probably processed differently after the first or second successive presentations. Furthermore, specific language-related neural activity may be unretrievable because it involves small amounts of neural tissue or because it is not synchronized to the stimulus presentation. In studies which have demonstrated language-related effects, the interpretation of results in accordance with linguistic theory is difficult because phonologic, semantic, and syntactic factors are generally confounded. Application of evoked potential and ERP techniques to uncover neural correlates of specific linguistic processes may, in fact, require studies using languages in which semantic and syntactic components are less intertwined than in English.

Development of the ERP

ERPs in infants, children, and even adolescents differ substantially from those elicited from adults. In infants, an ERP characterized by two high amplitude negative and positive waves, N_c and P_c, occur with latencies of about 700 and 1300 msec, respectively.[38] These ERPs are observed in response to both frequently and infrequently presented stimuli, although the wave amplitudes are greater following infrequent stimuli. N_c and P_c waves are present through the mid-teens, but progressively decrease in latency and amplitude as a function of age.[34] By age six, the N_c and P_c waves are elicited only by novel, unrecognizable stimuli.

P_3 waves to counted, infrequent signals have been observed in six-year-olds.[39] This is probably the youngest age at which one can expect reliable participation in the task. The latency and amplitude of the P_3 wave in young children is considerably greater than in adults. But both latency and amplitude progressively decrease as a function of age through the mid-teens.[34]

Developmental changes in ERPs, particularly the appearance and disappearance of N_c and P_c waves, suggest age-specific differences in cortical and neural mechanisms. An intriguing possibility is that the ERP changes parallel developmental changes in perceptual processing strategies. However, studies of cognitive development and ERP change are not yet available.

The P_3 latency to counted, infrequent signals continues to change throughout life. After reaching its minimum latency in the mid-teens, the P_3 latency then progressively increases through senescence.[40] The P_{3a}ERP to infrequent stimuli also increases in latency with age. In senile and presenile dementia, the rate of P_{3a} latency increase is rapidly accelerated and appears to parallel the course of the disease.[41] Unusually long P_{3a} latencies have also been associated with mental retardation.[4, 42] These findings suggest that the P_{3a} response may have some future application in the assessment of the cognitive status of children and adults.

CONCLUSIONS

The scalp-recorded evoked and event-related potentials provide the only available window through which to view operations of the human brain. However, much remains to be learned about the functions of neural activity underlying scalp-recorded potentials, and their relationship to hearing and language. Brain stem evoked potentials already provide a precise procedure for evaluating the integrity of auditory input structures. The later potentials show great promise for contributing to our understanding of higher cortical mechanisms and their development, and for assessment of cognitive and perceptual disorders. Whether or not this promise is fulfilled must await the results of future research.

REFERENCES

1. Jewett D, Williston J: Auditory evoked far fields averaged from the scalp of humans. Brain 94:681–696, 1971
2. Starr A, Achor LJ: Auditory brain stem responses in neurological disease. Arch Neurol 32:761–768, 1975
3. Stockard JJ, Rossiter VS: Clinical and pathologic correlates of brainstem auditory response abnormalities. Neurology 24:316–325, 1977
4. Galbraith GC, Squires N, Altair D, et al: Electrophysiological assessments in mentally retarded individuals: From brainstem to cortex, in Begleiter H (ed): Evoked Brain Potentials and Behavior. New York, Plenum, 1979, p 229
5. Don M, Eggermont JJ: Analysis of the click-evoked brainstem potentials in man using high-pass noise masking. J Acoust Soc Am 63:1084–1092, 1978
6. Yamada O, Toshiaki Y, Yamane H, et al: Clinical evaluation of the auditory evoked brain-stem response. ANL 2:97–105, 1975
7. Galambos R, Hecox K: Clinical applications of the human brainstem responses to auditory stimuli, in Desmedt JE (ed): Auditory Evoked Potentials in Man: Psychopharmalogical Correlates of Evoked Potentials. Basel, S. Karger, 1977, p1
8. Hecox K, Galambos R: Brainstem auditory evoked responses in human infants and adults. Arch Otolaryngol 99:30–33, 1974
9. Hecox K: Electrophysiological correlates of human auditory development, in Cohen LB, Salapateck P (eds): Infant Perception: From Sensation to Cognition, Vol 2. New York, Academic Press, 1975, p 151
10. Schulman-Galambos C, Galambos R: Brainstem auditory-evoked responses in premature infants. J Speech Hear Res 18:456–465, 1975
11. Picton TW, Hillyard SA, Krausz HI, et al: Human auditory evoked potentials I: Evaluation of components. Electroencephalogr Clin Neurophysiol 36:179–190, 1974
12. Starr A, Hamilton AE: Correlation between confirmed sites of neurological lesions and abnormalities of far-field auditory brainstem responses. Electroencephalogr Clin Neurophysiol 41:595–608, 1976
13. Buchwald JS, Huang C: Far field acoustic response: Origins in the cat. Science 189:382–384, 1975
14. Moushegian G, Rupert AL, Stillman RD: Scalp recorded early responses in man to frequencies in the speech range. Electroencephalogr Clin Neurophysiol 35:665–667, 1973
15. Stillman RD, Moushegian G, Rupert AL: Early tone-evoked responses in normal and hearing impaired subjects. Audiology 15:10–22, 1976
16. Moushegian G, Rupert AL, Stillman RD: Evaluation of frequency following potentials in man: Masking and clinical studies. Electroencephalogr Clin Neurophysiol 45:711–718, 1978

17. Huis n't Veld F, Osterhammel P, Terkildsen K: The frequency selectivity of the 500 Hz frequency following response. Scand Audiol 6:35–42, 1977
18. Stillman RD, Crow G, Moushegian G: Components of the frequency-following potential in man. Electroencephalogr Clin Neurophysiol 44:438–446, 1978
19. Gardi J, Merzenich M, McKean C: Origins of the scalp-recorded frequency-following response in the cat. Audiology 18:353–380, 1979
20. Gardi J, Salamy A, Mendelson T: Scalp-recorded frequency-following responses in neonates. Audiology 18:494–506, 1979
21. Celesia GG: Organization of auditory cortical areas in man. Brain 99:403–414, 1976
22. Ichikawa G, Kawamura S, Uchida T, et al: Nature of auditory evoked middle latency response. United States-Japanese Seminar on Auditory Responses from the Brain Stem, Honolulu, 1979, p14
23. Shinoda Y, Kaga K, Hink R: Origin of middle latency component in cats. United States-Japanese Seminar on Auditory Responses from the Brain Stem, Honolulu, 1979, p13
24. Mendel MI, Adkinson DC, Harker LA: Middle components of the auditory evoked potential in infants. Ann Otol Rhinol Laryngol 86:293–299, 1977
25. Wolf KE, Goldstein R: Middle component averaged electroencephalic responses to tonal stimuli from normal neonates. Arch Otolaryngol 104:508–513, 1978
26. Davis H, Davis PA, Loomis A: Electrical reactions of the human brain to auditory stimulation during sleep. J Neurophysiol 2:500–514, 1939
27. Picton TW, Woods DL, Baribeau-Braun J, et al: Evoked potential audiometry. J Otolaryngol 6:90–119, 1977
28. Davis H, Mast TE, Yoshie N: The slow response of the human cortex to auditory stimuli: Recovery processes. Electroencephalogr Clin Neurophysiol 21:105–113, 1966
29. Butler RA: The auditory evoked response to stimuli producing periodicity pitch. Psychophysiol 9:233–237, 1972
30. Davis H, Osterhammel PA, Wier CC, et al: Slow vertex potentials: Interactions among auditory, tactile, electric and visual stimuli. Electroencephalogr Clin Neurophysiol 33:537–545, 1972
31. Picton TW, Woods DL, Proulx GB: Human auditory sustained potentials, II: Stimulus relationships. Electroencephalogr Clin Neurophysiol 45:198–210, 1978
32. Picton TW, Hillyard SA: Human auditory evoked potentials, II: Effects of attention. Electroencephalogr Clin Neurophysiol 36:191–199, 1974
33. Ohlrich ES, Barnet AB, Weiss IP, et al: Auditory evoked potential development in early childhood: A longitudinal study. Electroencephalogr Clin Neurophysiol 44:411–423, 1978
34. Courchesne E: Neurophysiological correlates of cognitive development: Changes in long-latency event-related potentials from childhood to adulthood. Electroencephalogr Clin Neurophysiol 45:468–482, 1978
35. Cone B: The auditory evoked potential in the human neonate. Unpublished doctoral dissertation. University of Texas at Dallas, 1979
36. Squires NK, Squires KC, Hillyard SA: Two varieties of long-latency positive waves evoked by unpredictable auditory stimuli in man. Electroencephalogr Clin Neurophysiol 38:387–401, 1975
37. Courchesne E, Hillyard SA, Galambos R: Stimulus novelty, task relevance and the visual evoked potential in man. Electroencephalogr Clin Neurophysiol 39:131–143, 1975
38. Courchesne E, Ganz L, Norcia AM, et al: Long-latency event-related potentials in infants: Probability-dependent waves. Proceedings of the Seventh Annual Meeting of the Society for Neuroscience, Anaheim, 1977, p103
39. Courchesne E: Event-related brain potentials: Comparison between children and adults. Science 197:589–592, 1977

40. Goodin DS, Squires KC, Henderson BH, et al: Age-related variations in evoked potentials to auditory stimuli. Electroencephalogr Clin Neurophysiol 44:447–458, 1978

41. Squires K, Goodin D, Starr A: Event related potentials in development aging and dementia, in Lehmann D, Callaway E (eds): Human Evoked Potentials Application and Problems. New York, Plenum, 1979, p383

42. Squires NK, Galbraith GC, Aine CJ: Event related potential assessment of sensory and cognitive deficits in the mentally retarded, in Lehmann D, Callaway E (eds): Human Evoked Potentials Application and Problems. New York, Plenum, 1979, p397

BIBLIOGRAPHY

The following reviews and collections of research are recommended to the reader.

Begleiter H (ed): Evoked Brain Potentials and Behavior. New York: Plenum Press, 1979

Callaway E, Tueting P, Koslow SH (eds): Event-Related Brain Potentials in Man. New York: Academic Press, 1978

Gerber SE: Audiometry in Infancy. New York: Grune and Stratton, 1977

Lehmann D, Callaway E (eds): Human Evoked Potentials Applications and Problems. New York: Plenum Press, 1979

Picton TW, Woods DL, Baribeau-Braun J, et al: Evoked potential audiometry, J Otolaryngol 6:90–119, 1977

Regan D: Evoked Potentials in Psychology, Sensory Physiology and Clinical Medicine. London: Chapman and Hall, 1972

Stockard JJ, Stockard JE, Sharbrough FW: Nonpathologic factors influencing brainstem auditory evoked potentials. Am J EEG Technol 18:1–7–209, 1978

Patricia K. Kuhl

3

Infant Speech Perception: Reviewing Data on Auditory Category Formation

It has been almost a decade since the findings of Eimas *et al.*[1] on the human infant's responses to speech-sound stimuli were published. In this period, a considerable amount of data has been gathered on the perception of speech by young human infants. Based largely on the high-amplitude sucking technique,[1] the data demonstrate that very young normal infants (4 to 16 weeks of age) discriminate the acoustic cues underlying speech-sound distinctions in ways that can be described as "adult-like." That is, infants discriminate consonants that differ with respect to voicing[1] and place of articulation;[2, 3] they discriminate among fricatives[4] and liquids.[5] The tempo of spectral change, which for the adult is sufficient to cue a change in the manner of articulation, say from plosive to semivowel,[6] is also discriminable by the young infant.[7] Some of these contrasts have also been tested in the medial and final positions of syllables.[8-10] Trehub[11] demonstrated that infants discriminate between spectrally-dissimilar (/a/ vs /i/; /i/ vs /u/) vowels; Swoboda, Morse, and Leavitt[12] demonstrated that infants also discriminate between spectrally-similar vowels (/i/ vs /I/). The list of negative findings is relatively short. Other than for certain fricatives[13] and stimuli in which the discriminable contrast is embedded within the syllable (/atapa/ vs /ataba/; /mapa/ vs /pama/),[11] no negative findings for speech-sound contrasts that are phonemic in English have been reported, and no studies which attempt to replicate the above mentioned failures have been published.

One could summarize these data, then, as providing strong evidence that very young infants (one to four months of age) have sufficient auditory acuity to discriminate the acoustic differences which distinguish many, perhaps all, of the phonemic categories of English when they are represented by canonical consonant-vowel (CV) syllables. This is an important conclusion because if the infant's auditory capabilities were not sufficiently good to perceive the appropriate differences among stimuli, the infant would have an extremely difficult time attempting to learn language.

In addition to the ability to perceive the relevant *differences* between stimuli, however, the infant's attempts to learn language would be aided by the perception of *similarity* or *equivalence* between certain stimuli. To explain why the perception of similarity may be of interest, we have to develop a perspective on the formation of auditory categories.

CURRENT ISSUES: FORMATION OF AUDITORY CATEGORIES

Category Centers and Category Boundaries

A central theme in perceptual psychology relates to the study of perceptual groupings. Just as the field of vision has attempted to explain the perceptual recognition of patterns or of size and shape constancy, the field of audition has attempted to explain auditory pattern perception and speech-sound constancy. Each discipline has examined the extent to which changes in the physical parameters of a stimulus can be related to a change, or a lack of change, in its perceived attributes. Similarly, each field has been impressed (and baffled) by the difficulty involved in the identification of the critical stimulus information that underlies perceptual groupings, largely because of the extreme variation in the physical parameters of objects or events in the world that look or sound similar to a viewer or listener. In other words, the problem of perceptual similarity, or constancy, refers to the fact that viewers or listeners form perceptual categories, presumably based on a set of abstract dimensions of the physical stimulus, and do so despite the presence of many other dimensions that are prominent but irrelevant to the categorization process.

The study of categorization for speech sounds has focused on two rather different phenomena.[14] One approach has been the extensive work on the perception of the *boundaries* between categories indicative of studies on categorical perception. Studies of categorical perception involve a highly restricted and narrowly defined set of conditions for testing the discrimination and identification of stimuli.[15] They involve the use of computer-synthesized stimuli in which one set of acoustic cues considered to be sufficient to distinguish between two phonetic categories are varied in stepwise fashion to create a continuum of sounds; all other noncriterial dimensions, such as fundamental frequency, intensity, and duration, are held constant. The evidence for categorical perception derives from the fact that, under these testing conditions, listeners perceive all variants of the stimulus within the boundaries of a phoneme as the same, while the perception of differences between variants is maximal across phoneme boundaries.

The other approach has been to attempt to define the set of acoustic cues that underlie the perception of similarities (constancy) for any group of exemplars, all belonging to the same phonetic category. These studies involve the acoustic analysis of many different naturally produced or synthetically produced exemplars representing a category. In this approach, the noncriterial acoustic dimensions, such as the phonetic context, the position in an utterance, or the talker who utters the token, are allowed to vary, thus producing wide variation in the physical representations of the acoustic cues that are considered to be critical to a particular phonetic distinction.

Both of these approaches tap a listener's proclivity to form acoustic categories: categorical perception assesses the perceived discontinuities or boundaries between categories; perceptual constancy studies are aimed more at defining the category centers, the prototypes which best fit the description of the category. Categorical perception has been widely studied, but the study of constancy has been discouraged largely by a set of early descriptive studies which failed to identify invariant acoustic correlates to perceived categories.[16] Recent studies by Stevens and Blumstein,[17] Blumstein and Stevens,[18] and Searle, Jacobson and Rayment,[19] however, represent renewed interest in this approach. They have adopted the position that much of the difficulty that has been experienced in identifying invariant acoustic cues for phonetic categories stemmed from a lack of information concerning the way in which the peripheral auditory system transforms complex signals like speech. Thus, more recent approaches have relied on psychoacoustic data to create speech-analysis programs which mimic peripheral auditory processing. These cochlear-modeling approaches have been more successful in identifying invariant acoustic cues for speech sounds (see [20] for further review of these approaches to speech perception).

Data Obtained in Studies of Infant Speech Perception

CATEGORICAL PERCEPTION: THE STUDY OF CATEGORY BOUNDARIES

Categorical perception for speech sounds has been verified in adult listeners for many phonetic features.[16] The essential definition of categorical perception requires testing an adult listener's perceptual ability under two conditions: when stimuli from a computer-synthesized speech-sound continuum are presented singly for identification, and when they are presented in pairs for discrimination. The computer-synthesized continuum ranges from one speech sound to another (such as from /da/ to /ta/). Tokens constructed along the continuum are equidistant, that is, they vary equally from one another in the criterion dimension. The typical result of these studies is that the adult listener's perception is constrained in certain ways: first, an adult listener's discrimination performance for two speech sounds that were given the same phonetic label is near chance levels; second, the discrimination performance for stimuli that were labeled differently but are not further apart on the continuum than the previous pair, is nearly perfect. In other words, listeners perceive the differences between stimuli when they are given different phonetic labels but do not discriminate between them if they were not given different phonetic labels.

The early work on categorical perception demonstrated a distinct dichotomy between speech and nonspeech; speech was categorically perceived and nonspeech was not.[21] This phenomenon was thought to reflect the workings of a perceptual mechanism that responded only to the phonetic value of a speech sound, ignoring its precise acoustic details. More recently, however, clear demonstrations of categorical perception of acoustic continua that are not perceived as speech have been puolisned.[22-25] There can be no doubt that, given an appropriate continuum, these seemingly specific-to-speech results can be obtained with nonspeech stimuli. In addition, recent demonstrations show that changes in the discrimination of within-category speech-sound pairs (pairs discriminated at chance levels in the original paradigm) can be manipulated either by training[26] or by employing a discrimination procedure that reduces the degree to which the stimuli must be labeled and remembered.[27, 28]

The important role that categorical perception was thought to play in revealing the underlying operations of a speech-sound processor is evident from early writings on the subject.[15] It is not surprising, then, that the first work attempting to evaluate whether infant listeners demonstrated these same perceptual constraints was considered critical to the question of an infant's innate propensity for the perception of speech sounds, and the conclusion of early investigators of infant speech perception that infants process speech in a "linguistic mode".[29, 30]

METHODS FOR TESTING CATEGORICAL PERCEPTION IN INFANT LISTENERS

The high-amplitude-sucking (HAS) technique has been successfully used to study the infant's ability to discriminate speech-sound pairs. Briefly, a speech sound is presented to the infant each time he produces a sucking response whose amplitude exceeds a criterion. That particular speech sound is presented until the infant's sucking rate drops below some decrement criterion (habituation). Then, experimental infants are presented with a different speech sound while control infants continue to be presented with the first sound.

Figure 3-1 demonstrates the procedure. The infant sucks on a blind nipple attached to a pressure transducer. The infant's sucking responses produce pressure changes inside the nipple that are monitored with a standard pressure transducer. The resulting pressure waveforms are shown at the bottom of the figure; an amplitude criterion is set for each infant during a "no-sound" baseline condition. After the baseline level has been established, a speech sound (typically 500 msec in duration) is presented immediately after each response with a maximum repetition rate of one per second.

A typical experimental and control infant's data are shown in Figure 3-2. The abscissa is labeled in minutes before and after the "shift point" (the point at which the sound is changed for experimental infants). During the first minute of contingent sound presentation, the response rate typically decreases. Most infants appear startled and stop sucking for a moment when the first sounds are presented, as suggested by the decrease in response rate between the baseline minute and the first minute of sound presentation. Eventually, however, the response rate increases and reaches a maximum. The same speech sound is presented until a 20 percent decrement in response rate occurs for two consecutive minutes. When this habituation criteria is met, infants in the experimental group are presented with a new sound while infants in the control group continue to hear the first sound. Both the experimental and the control infants are monitored for four minutes after the habituation criterion is met. The mean response rate for the two minutes immediately preceding the shift is subtracted from the mean response rate for the two minutes immediately following the shift to obtain a difference score for each infant. Experimental infants typically increase their response rates when the speech sound is changed (dishabituation) while control infants, who are presented with the same sound, either continue to decrease or do not change their response rates. Significant differences between the two groups of infants is taken as evidence that the infants can discriminate the two speech sounds.

Nearly ten years have passed since Siqueland and Delucia[31] described the HAS technique. Since that time, much debate has ensued over the typical pattern of results that are obtained. When many laboratories utilize the same or nearly the same technique, quite a few investigations are aimed at simply understanding why the technique works as it does. Kuhl and Miller[32] demonstrated that the typical increase in sucking responses both at the onset of the experiment and after habituation did not occur for a "no-sound" control group. Trehub and Chang[33] demonstrated that the sound must be presented contingently on the high-amplitude sucking responses rather than noncontingently in order to demonstrate the dramatic increase between baseline and maximum. Williams and Golenski[34] demonstrated a similar necessity for

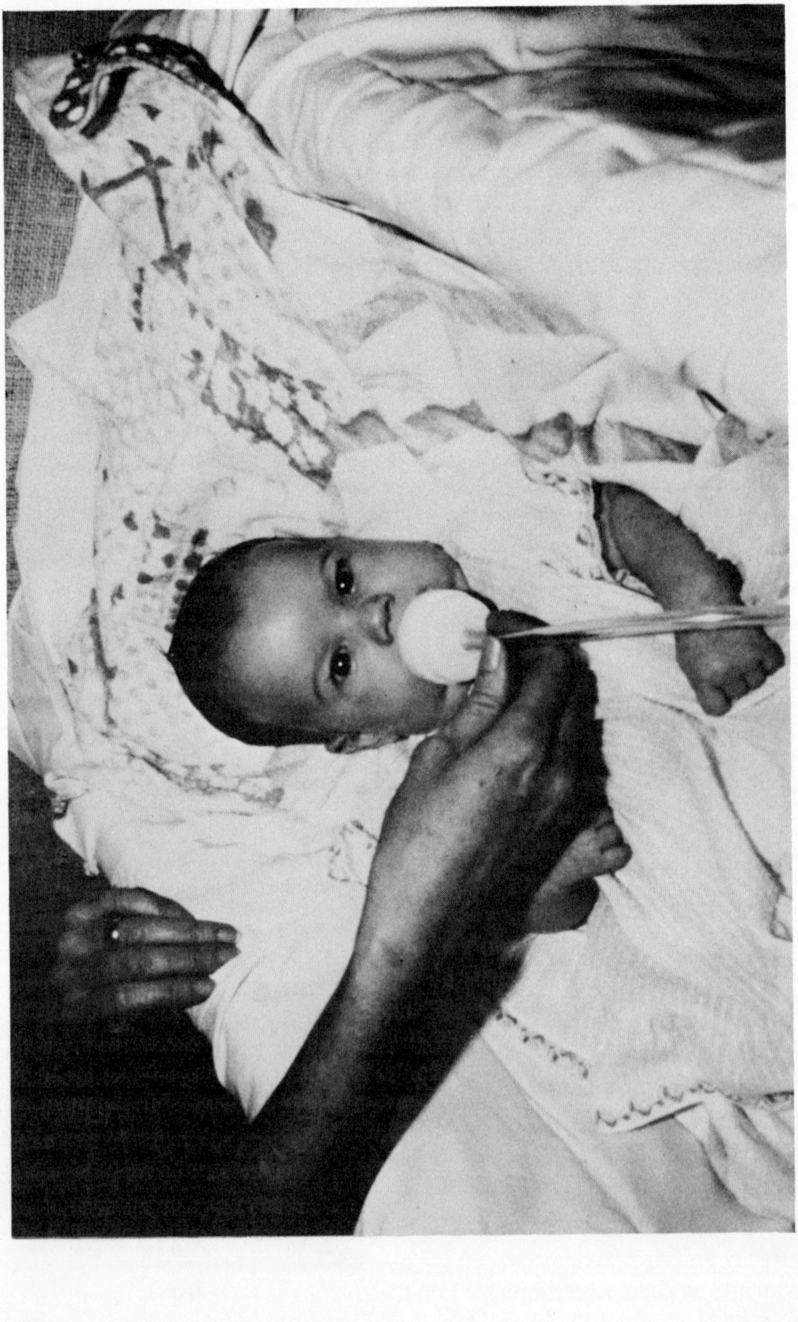

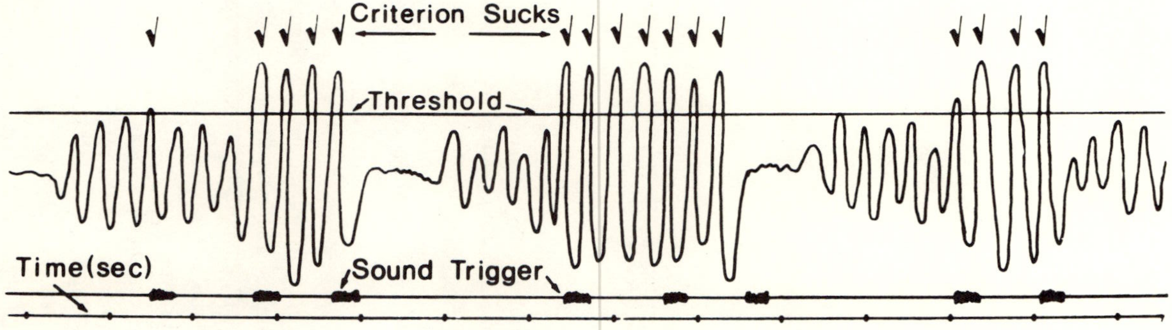

Fig. 3-1. Eight-week-old infant sucking on a "blind" nipple to produce speech sounds. Pressure changes resulting from the infant's sucking responses are monitored and those sucking responses which exceed an amplitude criterion (labeled "threshold") are defined as "criterion" responses; criterion responses trigger a speech-sound presentation with a maximum repetition rate of one per second. (Reprinted from Kuhl PK: Speech perception in early infancy: The acquisition of speech-sound categories, in Hirsh SK, Eldredge DH, Hirsh IJ, Silverman SR (Eds.): Hearing and Davis: Essays Honoring Hallowell Davis. St. Louis: Washington University Press, 1976.)

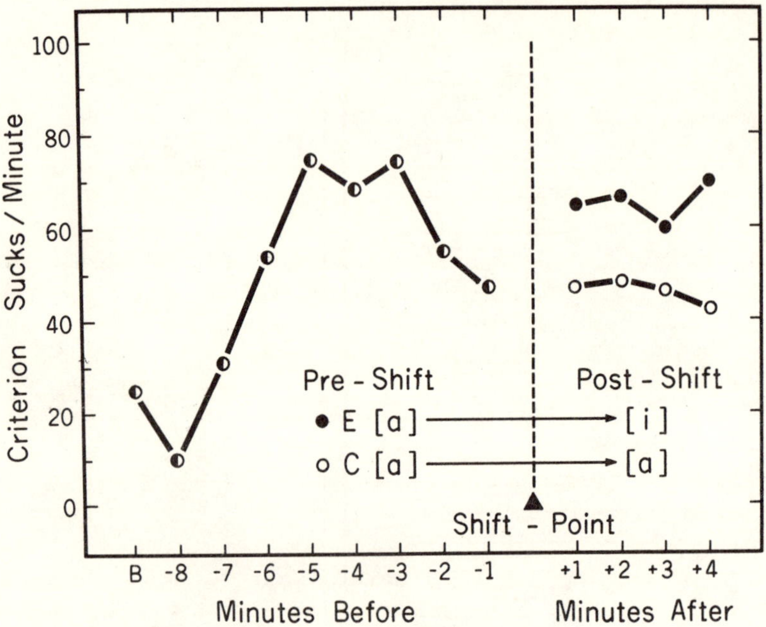

Fig. 3-2. Minute-by-minute criterion sucking responses for one experimental and one control infant; responses are averaged for the preshift period. (Reprinted from Kuhl PK: Speech perception in early infancy: The acquisition of speech-sound categories in Hirsh SK, Eldredge DH, Hirsh IJ, Silverman SR (Eds.): Hearing and Davis: Essays Honoring Hallowell Davis. St. Louis: Washington University Press, 1976.)

contingent sound presentation in order to obtain a reliable increase in sucking responses when the sound is changed. These results, along with the fact that many laboratories, each with small unavoidable modifications in the technique, have produced similar results, argues that the technique works on the principle of a conditioned operant response.

The technique, however, has certain drawbacks. The fact that the speech sound serves as both the discriminative and the reinforcing stimulus make it difficult to interpret negative results; it is impossible to separate the infant's inability to discriminate the two sounds from his lack of interest in them. In addition, only group data can be obtained. Sucking responses are under the control of many diverse factors and the pattern of responses is not shown by each and every infant. A third problem involves the high attrition rates (50 to 60 percent). Fourth, the technique works best for infants under four months of age. At older ages, infants become restless in infant seats and are not, in general, as interested in sucking continuously on a nipple.

DATA OBTAINED IN CATEGORICAL PERCEPTION EXPERIMENTS WITH INFANTS

While infant listeners cannot provide labels for stimuli in an experiment, they can be tested in a discrimination paradigm such as that provided by the HAS technique just described. Studies in which pairs of stimuli were drawn from a synthetic speech-sound continuum demonstrated that infants discriminated two stimuli when they were labeled differently by adult listeners, but did not discriminate between stimuli that were labeled similarly by adult listeners. These data were taken as support for the notion that infants perceived the synthetic-speech stimuli in ways that resembled the categorical perception demonstrated in adult listeners. These findings were first shown for a voiced-voiceless (/ba-pa/) continuum;[1] subsequently the same results have been demonstrated for a place of articulation (/dae-gae/) continuum[3] and a liquid (/ra-la/) continuum.[5]

These studies lead to the conclusion that, like adult listeners, infant listeners are particularly sensitive to small differences between sound stimuli, particularly when those differences serve to separate adult-defined phonetic categories. That infants should do so is extremely relevant to their linguistic development since the infant appears to perceive a natural perceptual discontinuity between acoustic events that will come to signal significant (meaningful) differences between words.

One of the important questions not answered sufficiently by the data is whether an infant at some early age demonstrates these perceptual discontinuities for *all* phonetic distinctions, even those not relevant to the linguistic environment in which he is being raised. If it were the case that the infant demonstrated the effect for a universal set of phonetic distinctions, then one would argue that due to the lack of exposure to certain phonetic units (those phonetic units not utilized by the language) during development, the infant somehow loses the ability to distinguish them as contrasting phonetic elements.[35] In other words, this line of inquiry suggests that infants have innate mechanisms enabling them to perceive all the possible phonetic distinctions of natural languages. In the course of development, however, they lose the ability to perceive contrasts not relevant to their language community while maintaining the ability to distinguish among those that are relevant to the language they eventually will learn.

This is a complex issue because it requires, first, the demonstration that very young infants, regardless of their linguistic environments, behave similarly —demonstrating these boundary effects for contrasts that are used in their linguistic environments and for other contrasts, that are not used in their environments. Second, this theoretic posture requires the demonstration that infants from different linguistic environments behave differently at some later point in time, demonstrating an effect of linguistic exposure. While the data gathered to date loosely support such claims, they are not without contradiction. The evidence is fairly convincing that infants under four months of age, reared in non-English-speaking environments, are capable of discriminating at least one phonetic contrast (voiceless unaspirated /pa/ from voiceless aspirated /p^ha/) that is phonemic in English but not in the infant's native language. Streeter[36] demonstrated that two-month-old African Kikuyu infants discriminated the English contrast, in addition to discriminating a voicing contrast that is phonemic in the Kikuyu language but not in English (prevoiced /ba/ from voiceless unaspirated /pa/). Lasky, Syrdal-Lasky, and Klein[37] demonstrated similar results for Spanish infants using a heart-rate technique to measure responses.

However, the case for discrimination of the prevoiced /ba/ from the voiceless unaspirated /pa/ by American infants under four months of age is not quite as clear. Eimas[35] failed to provide evidence that American infants discriminated pairs of stimuli that are as close on the continuum as those discriminated by the Spanish and Kikuyu infants. As Kuhl and Miller[38] note, however, there are a number of problems with these cross-language comparisons. First, the stimuli are synthesized to manipulate an acoustic cue that is acoustically fragile, and is likely to be subject to variation due to the differences in acoustic calibration across laboratories. A recent set of studies applied this approach to the study of older infants. Using the head-turn technique, Eilers, Wilson, and Moore[39] and Eilers, Gavin, and Wilson[40] tested six-month-old American and Spanish infants in the same laboratory and demonstrated that while both groups perceived the English contrast, only the Spanish infants discriminated the Spanish contrast.

Eilers, Gavin, and Wilson[40] would attribute the superiority of the Spanish infants on the Spanish contrast at six months of age to linguistic exposure, but, in the absence of data demonstrating that American infants do discriminate the contrast at an earlier age (say, under four months of age), the story is far from complete. Using a more sensitive technique, Aslin and colleagues[41] showed that six-month-old American infants do discriminate the Spanish contrast. But, to date they have not tested Spanish infants to see if the Spanish infants would in some way demonstrate a superior ability to do so by six months of age.

In summary, both the demonstrations of similar perceptual tendencies by very young infants from different linguistic environments, and the demonstrations of increasingly dissimilar perceptual tendencies by older infants from different linguistic environments (presumably due to linguistic exposure), are incomplete. These areas will remain important target areas of research in the future.

Perceptual Constancy: The Study of Perceptual Similarity

GENERAL CONSIDERATIONS

However extensive the data on speech-sound perception by infants may be, we have little information concerning an infant's perception of phonetic similarity for phonemes which appear in different phonetic contexts, appear in different positions in a syllable, or are spoken by different talkers. We might expect this kind of task to present quite a different set of problems for the infant than the typical discrimination task. Gibson[42] describes perceptual constancy as involving at least two processes. First, a listener must discover and focus on the acoustic dimension relevant to the particular phonetic distinction. This may be relatively easy when the phonetic context and the talker are held constant as in the typical experiments described above in which single tokens from each of two phonetic categories were to be discriminated.[1-4, 11, 13] But when a variety of tokens representing a phonetic distinction are used, the critical cues vary and the listener must abstract a cue that is common to the set. One would predict from this that the discovery of a set of abstract configurational properties or attributes that typify a phonetic category would depend upon the appropriate or sufficient exposure to a set of exemplars of that phonetic category, exemplars that differ with respect to phonetic context and talker.

The second process related to the perception of constancy is a concomitant of the first. When the phonetic context and the talker are varied, acoustically-prominent but phonetically irrelevant acoustic dimensions are introduced. For the infant to recognize that /di/ and /du/ are somehow similar, he must ignore the most prominent difference between them, that is, the vowel. The fundamental frequency and timbre differences between the voices of different talkers, and the pitch contour of the utterances, are other prominent acoustic characteristics that a listener must ignore when categorizing phonetically since these dimensions do not provide critical information concerning the phonetic identification of the stimulus.

These two processes—abstracting the critical dimensions that typify a phonetic category and, at the same time, ignoring other prominent but irrelevant dimensions—have been discussed in the literature on visual perception. There is some evidence in this literature to suggest that some aspects of these two processes are learned. It has been shown, for example, that infants become increasingly adept at focusing their attention on the critical aspects of a stimulus array. A study of eye movements, directed at an unfamiliar design that must be remembered demonstrated that three-year-olds keep their eyes fixed on a single spot longer and do not systematically explore figures, while six-year-olds orient to the distinctive features employing brief and frequent gazes and systematically exploring the figure.[43] Vurpillot[44] studied the eye movements of children between five and nine years of age in a same-different comparison task. The data from the study supported the notion that skill in scanning systematically and in sampling the relevant features increases with age.

The notion that infants become increasingly selective in their visual attention carries with it the implication that infants become more adept at filtering out irrelevant information. Evidence from experiments on incidental learning support this notion. Gibson[42] reported experiments run by herself and colleagues on form identification in five-year-old preschoolers. The task was simply to learn the names of nine roman-capital letters of the alphabet. When presented during the learning sessions, the letters were colored—three were red, three blue, and three yellow; these colors, of course, did not differentiate the letters uniquely, but served as an irrelevant dimension. After practice sessions, the children were asked to identify the same nine forms that were now colored black. In addition, they were tested for recall of the color of each of the forms. Gibson reported that the children remembered correctly as many, or more, colors than they did the names of the letters, even though color was an irrelevant dimension in this experiment. The experiment was repeated with nine-year-olds using artificial graphemes rather than letters. The task was identical. For these children, recall of the names of the graphemes had improved slightly; but more importantly, color was recalled at a level no better than chance. Some children did not even remember what colors had been presented. In a related experiment, Maccoby and Hagen[45] presented six picture cards, each with a distinctively colored background, to first through seventh grade children. Subjects were instructed to remember the order of the colors presented. After repeated trials on color identification, the subjects were asked to recall the picture that had appeared on each one of the colors. The results demonstrated that recall on the main task increases steadily with age, but that first through fifth graders recalled the correct picture significantly more than than seventh graders, even though it was an irrelevant dimension.

In summary, Gibson concludes that there is evidence to suggest that the ability to seek out the invariant information in a stimulus array is a developmental phenomenon. Both the tendency for greater efficiency at picking up the invariant information in a stimulus array, as well as the increasing tendency to filter out irrelevant information, contributes to this gradual approach to perceptual economy.

TWO EARLY STUDIES

Only recently have researchers attempted to find out whether infants are capable of recognizing the similarity among sounds that have the same phonetic label when the sounds occur in different phonetic contexts, occur in different positions in a syllable, or are spoken by different talkers. Fodor, Garrett, and Brill[46] examined the acquisition of a head-turn response for visual reinforcement in 14- to 18-week-old infants under two stimulus conditions. In both conditions, three syllables were randomly presented (/pi/, /ka/, /pu/) but only two of the three were reinforced. In one condition, the stimuli being reinforced were phonetically related (/pi/ and /pu/); in the other condition, the stimuli being reinforced were not phonetically related (/pi/ and /ka/). The hypothesis tested was as follows: if infants tend to hear the similarity between two syllables that begin with the same consonant, in spite of the differences in the acoustic cues for that consonant and in spite of the irrelevant differences between the two syllables that must be ignored (like their vowels), then their tendencies to learn the association ought to differ in the two conditions. The results showed that the proportion of head turns obtained from the infants when phonetically similar sounds were reinforced was significantly greater than the proportion of head turns obtained when phonetically dissimilar sounds were reinforced.

These data demonstrated that the infants grouped the syllables beginning with /p/ more readily than they grouped the syllables that did not share a phonetic feature. But the data also demonstrated that neither task was accomplished very accurately. Two factors may have made the task inordinately difficult. First, observations in our own laboratory on the audiometric testing of infants has demonstrated to us that until 5½ months of age, a large percentage of infants do not make volitional head-turn responses for a visual reinforcer with ease. At 5½ months or older, infants make head-turn responses easily and 90 to 95 percent of the infants are conditionable when an easy contrast (/a/ vs /i/) is tested. Second, the task was very difficult; it involved a two-response differentiation. That is, a head turn either to the right or to the left was required (two different responses) depending on the loudspeaker from which the reinforced stimulus was presented.

Kuhl and Miller[32] began a systematic exploration of the infant's predispositions to form acoustic categories that were based on shared phonetic features. The perception of vowel categories seemed an appropriate place to begin. The earliest descriptions of the acoustic cues which govern vowel identity were relatively straightforward. Vowel perception is directly related to the location of formants on the frequency axis, and two or three formants are sufficient to computer-synthesize the full complement of English vowels.[47] However, in natural speech, the vowel nucleus is coarticulated with one or more consonants and, in rapid speech, a steady-state value is rarely achieved.[48] In addition, the acoustic properties of the vowel nucleus are influenced by the coarticulated consonants.[49, 50] Assuming a constant vocal tract length, the formant frequencies directly reflect the resonances created as the configuration of the vocal tract changes for different vowels.[51] But most importantly, a dramatic variation in formant frequency occurs when the overall dimensions of the vocal tract are changed. Thus, when the identical vowel is produced by a male, a female, and a child, the formant frequencies are quite different.[52] Furthermore, these changes in overall vocal tract dimensions, such as vocal tract length, are not proportional[53] so that the resulting formant frequencies are not related in a multiplicative way such as in the transposition of a melody.[54] Fant[55] has demonstrated that the scale factor relating the formants produced by a male, a female, and a child is not constant across vowels or across formants within a particular vowel. In other words, there is no constant relationship between the formants spoken by different talkers. Still, formant locations can be described as the invariant cues which allow the adult listener to perceive the similarity among vowels.

These facts led a number of theorists to hypothesize that listeners perceive vowel identity by calibrating or normalizing each utterance, that is, by referencing it to a coordinate system based on that talker's extreme articulations.[56-58] Experimental tests of the notion that listeners require exposure to a talker's "calibrating vowels" in order to correctly identify other vowels spoken by that talker have not been supported.[59] In fact, there is no evidence that the identification of vowels can be improved by presenting the calibrating vowels prior to the target vowel.[60] Our understanding of how vowels are perceived remains unclear.

As a preliminary step toward testing perceptual constancy in infants, Kuhl and Miller[32] asked whether 4- to 16-week-old infants could detect a change in a target dimension if an irrelevant dimension was randomly varied throughout the experiment, serving as a kind of distracting stimulus. The high-amplitude-sucking paradigm was employed. A change in the target dimension occurred at the shift-point, but the irrelevant dimension was randomly varied throughout both the pre- and post-shift periods.

In one condition, the target dimension was a phonemic change in the vowel and the irrelevant dimension was the pitch contour of the vowel; in a second condition, the target dimension was the pitch contour of the vowel and the irrelevant dimension was the vowel color. The choice of pitch contour as a distracting acoustic dimension is particularly appropriate given that the literature is replete with suggestions that suprasegmental dimensions such as pitch contour, loudness and stress pattern are more salient than segmental (phonetic) dimensions at this young age.[61] The stimuli were two /a/s and two /i/s synthesized such that one /a/ and one /i/ had identical monotone pitch contours, and one /a/ and one /i/ had identical rise-fall pitch contours. Discrimination of vowel color and pitch contour targets was tested *with* and *without* irrelevant variation (distracting stimulus) in the other dimension.

The data demonstrated that infants detected a vowel change, that is, discriminated the two vowels, regardless of the distraction imposed by the random changes in the pitch contour of the vowels. In contrast, infants detected a change in the pitch contour of the vowel only when all other dimensions were held constant; they failed to respond to a pitch contour change when the vowel color was randomly changed. In addition, infants responded for a significantly longer period of time before habituating (pre-shift) when the vowel color was constantly changing than when the pitch contour was constantly changing. Using these stimuli, it would appear that the vowel-color dimension captured the infant's attention more readily than the pitch contour, both when pitch contour was the target and when it served as the distractor. This research demonstrated the infant's ability to tolerate some degree of distraction and still make the phonetic discrimination, but it did not demonstrate the infant's ability to recognize the phonetic similarity among vowel tokens when the talker producing the vowels was varied. Furthermore, this study did not support the notion that suprasegmental dimensions are more salient at this age.

In order to extend these results to a situation in which the infant had to contend with variation in both the critical and noncritical dimensions of the signals, Kuhl[62] combined the use of a head-turn technique for visual reinforcement with an experimental format that required the infant to recognize the similarity among tokens in a category. Research using this format is described below.

METHODS FOR TESTING AUDITORY CATEGORY FORMATION WITH INFANTS: THE HEAD-TURN TECHNIQUE

Many laboratories have attempted to develop a head-turn technique for use in speech-sound discrimination testing but, until recently, no one had described a technique that had been extensively tested and found to work with a large number of infants. This technique was originally developed for assessing auditory thresholds by a team of clinical audiologists at the University of Washington in Seattle.[63] Later, the technique was adapted by Eilers, Wilson, and Moore[13] to study speech-sound discrimination. In the Eilers, Wilson, and Moore study, infants were trained to make a head turn whenever a speech sound, repeated once every second as a background stimulus, was changed to a comparison speech sound. A head turn which occurred during the presentation of the comparison stimulus was rewarded with the presentation of a visual stimulus, for example, a toy monkey that would clap cymbals when activated.

Two types of trials, change trials and control trials, are run. During a change trial, the stimulus is actually changed from one speech sound to another speech sound for the duration of the observation interval (typically 4 to 6 seconds). During control trials of the same length, the sound is not changed. For both types of trials, the experimenter and the assistant report whether or not a head turn has occurred during the specified observation interval. If both judges report that a head turn has occurred on a change trial, the trial is scored as correct; if one or neither reports ahead turn, an error is scored. During a control trial, if either judge reports a head turn, the trial is scored as an error; if neither report a head turn, the trial is scored as correct. Eilers, Wilson, and Moore[13] accepted a criterion of at least five out of six correct responses in six consecutive trials, half of which were change trials and half of which were control trials, as evidence that the infant discriminated the comparison stimulus from the background.

The experimental-control suite is shown in Figure 3-3. The infant is held

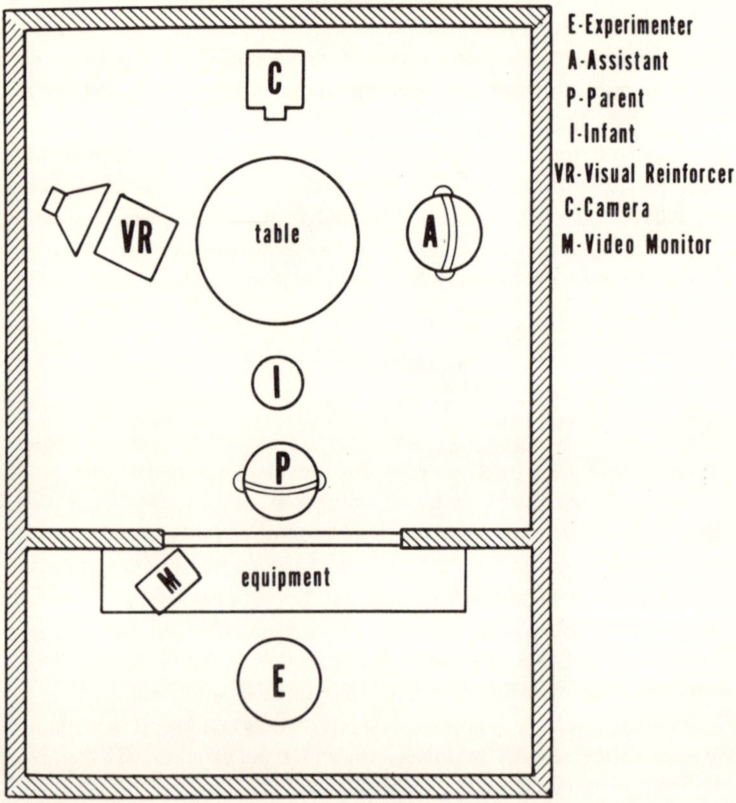

Fig. 3-3. Experimental/control suite for the head-turn experiments. The reinforcer is located at 90° to the left of the assistant, approximately five feet from the infant. (Reprinted from Kuhl PK: Speech perception in early infancy: Perceptual constancy for spectrally dissimilar vowel categories. J Acoust Soc Am 66:1668–1679, 1979, with permission.)

by a parent so that he faces an assistant. The assistant maintains the infant's attention at midline or directly in front by manipulating a variety of silent toys. A loudspeaker is located at a 90° azimuth to the assistant; the visual reinforcer is placed directly in front of the loudspeaker. A toy animal is housed in a dark plexiglass box so that the animal is not visible until the lights mounted inside the box are illuminated. The experimenter is housed in an adjoining control room which contains a tape deck and a logic device. The two speech sounds being tested are stored on two separate channels and on each channel the sound repeats once every 1 to 2 seconds, depending on the specific experiment.

This basic technique has been improved in two ways since it was originally described.[13] First, the logic device controlling the experiment is more sophisticated. In a recent modification of the technique,[62] the logic device contains a probability generator; the state of the probability generator determines whether a change trial or a control trial will be run. In this way, when the experimenter begins a trial by depressing a start button, he has no control over the type of trial that will be run. This ensures that the experimenter cannot inadvertently (or otherwise) start change trials when the infant is visually engaged by the toys. The logic device also times the trial interval, records both the experimenter's and the assistant's votes, scores the trial, activates the reinforcer when it is appropriate, records the latency of the infant's head-turn response, and prints all of the above data for each trial. This automatic recording system allows one to assess the agreement of the two judges.

The second improvement in the technique consists of a number of added experimental controls, in addition to those necessitated by the change in the logic, which improve the validity of technique. This improvement[7, 41, 62] requires that both the mother and the assistant wear headphones and listen to music throughout the session; the intensity level of the music is adjusted to mask the stimulus change. In this way, neither the mother nor the assistant can differentially change their behavior during change or control trials. Mothers do not know when trials occur. The assistant is informed that a trial is occurring by a small vibrating pin that is located on the vote button held in the assistant's hand, but he is unaware of the type of trial. These added controls achieve a situation in which both the mother and the assistant are "blind," and the experimenter does not know ahead of time what type of trial, change or control, will be run.

The technique has been successfully employed with infants as young as 5½ months[63] and as old as 18 months of age.[13] It is ideally suited to infants in the 5½- to 10-month age range. Beyond this age, infants tend to be increasingly restless, and they become wise with regard to object permanence. That is, the 10-month-old appears to realize that the monkey is still in the box, even if the lights are out and it cannot be seen; this causes the infant to want to peer in the box. For a six-month-old, the notion, out of sight and out of mind, still appears to hold.

Recently, Kuhl[62] adapted the basic technique just described to test auditory category formation in infants. In this adaptation of the technique, Kuhl systematically increased the number of tokens in both the background and the comparison categories in progressive stages of an experiment. In this experiment, the infant was required to achieve 90 percent correct performance (nine out of ten consecutive trials, half of which are change trials and half of which are control trials) at each stage before advancing to the next stage. The extent to which the infant's learned responses to single tokens from a phonetic category generalized to novel tokens from the same phonetic category, was evidence that the infant recognized the similarity among speech tokens sharing a common phonetic feature despite the many ways in which the tokens differed acoustically.

Table 3-1 describes the stimuli in the background category and in the

Table 3-1.
Stimulus Ensembles for the Background and Comparison Categories for All Five Stages of the /a/ vs /i/ Experiment (The talker and pitch contour values for each stimulus are given in parentheses)*

	Experimental Stages	
	Background	Comparison
Conditioning	/a/ (Male, fall)	/i/ (Male, fall)
Initial Training	/a/ (Male, fall)	/i/ (Male, fall)
Pitch Variation	/a/ (Male, fall) /a/ (Male, rise)	/i/ (Male, fall) /i/ (Male, rise)
Talker Variation	/a/ (Male, fall) /a/ (Female, fall)	/i/ (Male, fall) /i/ (Female, fall)
Talker × Pitch Variation	/a/ (Male, fall) /a/ (Male, rise) /a/ (Female, fall) /a/ (Female, rise)	/i/ (Male, fall) /i/ (Male, rise) /i/ (Female, fall) /i/ (Female, rise)
Entire Ensemble	/a/ (Male, fall) /a/ (Male, rise) /a/ (Female, fall) /a/ (Female, rise) /a/ (Child, fall) /a/ (Child, rise)	/i/ (Male, fall) /i/ (Male, rise) /i/ (Female, fall) /i/ (Female, rise) /i/ (Child, fall) /i/ (Child, rise)

*Reprinted from Kuhl PK: Speech perception in early infancy: Perceptual constancy for spectrally dissimilar vowel categories. J Acoust Soc Am 66:1668–1679, 1979, with permission.

comparison category for each of five stages in the /a/ vs /i/ category formation experiment.[62] In each category, the number of vowels is increased until the two ensembles include six different tokens spoken by three different talkers (male, female, and child) each with two different pitch contours (rise and rise-fall). In the initial training stage of the experiment, each of the two categories is represented by a single token; these two tokens are matched in every detail except for the critical cues which differentiate the two categories. In stage two, the pitch contour of the vowels in both categories is randomly changed from rise to rise-fall. The pitch-contour variation stage was included for two reasons: first, this stage could provide the infant with a cognitive set regarding the rules of this experimental "game." That is, category formation requires a certain mental set; the infant has to recognize that he is to group stimuli together based on their similarities, even though the stimuli differ in acoustically prominent ways. The pitch-contour variation ought to provide this mental set, and also serve as proof that the infant is capable of auditory category formation. A failure to generalize to new talkers, than, could not be attributed to an inability to form auditory categories.

In stage three, the talker producing the vowels is randomly varied between the male voice and the female voice. In stage four, both talkers produce the vowels with a randomly changing pitch contour. In the final stage, the child's voice (computer-synthesized), also with pitch-contour variations, is added to the ensemble bringing the total number of tokens in each category to six (three talkers × two pitch contours).

The criterion for progressing from one stage of the experiment to the next is nine out of ten consecutive trials correct, five of which are change trials and five of which are control trials. No more than three trials of one kind (either change or control) are allowed to occur consecutively. Typically, 25 trials are run each day in a 20-minute session. However, sessions were always terminated when an infant began to fuss or not attend to the assistant's toys. If, on the other hand, an infant was doing well, the session was extended. Infants were tested on consecutive days whenever that was possible.

The data resulting from this /a/ vs /i/ category-formation task[62] can be seen in Table 3-2. The number of trials to reach criterion performance is shown for four subjects. The data demonstrate that fairly rapid acquisition of the head-turning response occurred; all four subjects met the conditioniong criterion within the first 22 trials. Second, and more importantly, the infants demonstrated rapid transfer of learning from the training token to the novel exemplars of /a/ and /i/, the conditons of pitch, talker, and pitch × talker variation.

In a second experiment reported by Kuhl,[62] six-month-old infants were trained on the /a/ and /i/ tokens produced by the male talker, and then immediately presented with each of the novel tokens in the category. These data are

Table 3-2.
Trials to Criterion for Each Condition of the /a/ vs /i/ Experiment
(The session in which the criterion was met is listed in parentheses)

Condition	S_1	S_2	S_3	S_4	$\overline{X}$
Conditioning	12(1)	13(1)	5(1)	9(1)	9.75
Initial Training	23(2)	14(1)	32(2)	13(1)	20.50
Pitch Variation	11(2)	11(2)	10(2)	15(1)	11.75
Talker Variation	10(3)	10(2)	10(2)	14(2)	11.00
Talker × Pitch Variation	10(4)	29(3)	10(3)	18(2)	16.75
Entire Ensemble	10(4)	29(4)	22(4)	19(3)	20.00
Total Trials to Complete	76	106	89	88	89.75
Total Days to Complete	4	4	4	3	3.75

Reprinted from Kuhl PK: Speech perception in early infancy: Perceptual constancy for spectrally dissimilar vowel categories. J Acoust Soc Am 66:1668–1679, 1979, with permission.

shown for eight subjects in Figure 3-4. The histograms represent the percentage of head-turn responses that were made to each of the tokens in the reinforced category (either /a/ or /i/). The data demonstrate that the infants produced reliable head-turn responses to each of the tokens in the reinforced category (either /a/ or /i/). The data also demonstrate that the infants produced reliable head-turn responses to each of the novel tokens in the category.

Other examples of category formation for phonetic categories include the studies of fricative categories, such as /sa/ vs /ʃa/,[64] and categories based on a suprasegmental acoustic cue, pitch contour.[65]

DISCUSSION

General Comments

These results on the perception of constancy by young normal infants demonstrate their capability to recognize the abstract dimensions of sound in a task that has a considerable cognitive load. In order to complete the task, the infant must be capable of abstracting a similarity between the two phonetic units even though the acoustic components of the exemplars are not identical. In addition to abstracting this similarity, the infant must ignore very prominent but irrelevant dimensions such as pitch contour, talkers, and vowel context, as well as constantly monitor the signal and recall the rules of the game (something like, "turn to see the monkey when the sound changes from /a/ to /i/, no matter who says it or how it is said").

The advantages of this testing format are obvious. Since the multidimensional stimulus sets can be grouped according to a number of dimensions,

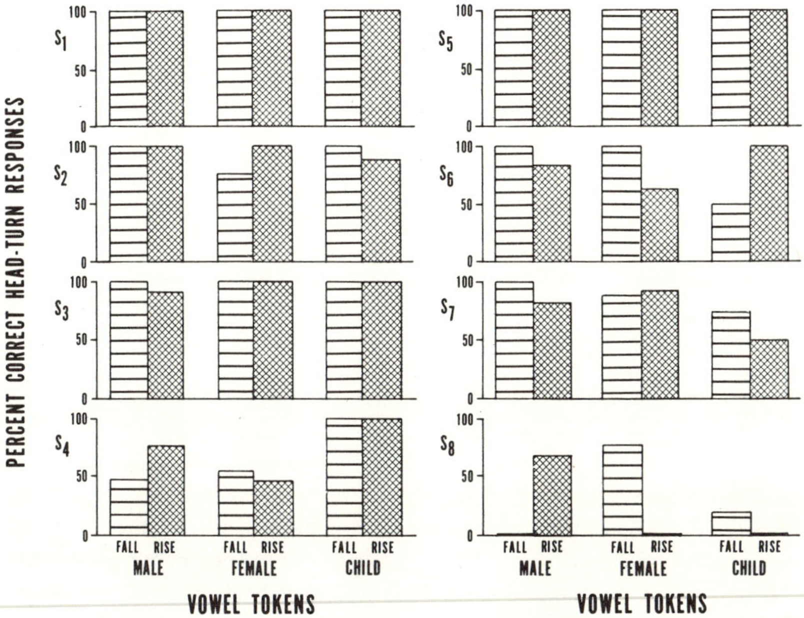

Fig. 3-4. Individual-subject data representing the percentage of correct head-turn responses which occurred during all change trials for each of the six stimuli presented during the /a/ vs /i/ category-formation experiment. (Reprinted from Kuhl PK: Speech perception in early infancy: Perceptual constancy for spectrally dissimilar vowel categories. J Acoust Soc Am 66:1668–1679, 1979, with permission.)

including segmental (vowel color, for example) as well as suprasegmental (intonation contour, for example) features, one can test the relative ease or efficiency an infant displays at forming acoustic categories based on these dimensions. In this way, one can assess their relative acoustic salience and determine whether an infant's auditory proclivities to form categories change with maturation and/or exposure to a particular language. In essence, this technique for studying category formation allows one to identify the infant's "sorting rules" for the separation of auditory stimuli.

Clinical Applications

While there are not data to suggest that an infant's skills at the formation of auditory categories is predictive of later language development, it may be a worthwhile investigation. It is important to note that the tasks used in these experiments require some cognitive sophistication as well as specific auditory attention and memory. The fact that the infant has to isolate and attend to some criterial acoustic information that is used to sort or categorize the stimuli, while ignoring other prominent auditory events, makes it likely that skill at the task is related to general measures of intelligence as well as auditory perception. The degree to which these skills are specifically correlated with language skills is simply unknown at this time.

The infants tested to date are considered to be developing normally—that is, they were not premature or in any way considered to be neurologically at risk and they have no familial history of hearing loss or positive history of middle-ear infection—yet they display varying skills in performing these tasks. Taken as a whole, the infants tested in category-formation studies of this type can be described as falling into one of three groups. Approximately 60 percent of the infants we have seen perform the tasks very well; they learn quickly and generalize easily. These infants are easy to train because an assistant learns quickly what kinds of toys capture the infant's attention, and the infant behaves in a consistent and predictable fashion. Another 30 percent of the infants are trainable but they require a greater number of trials to meet criterion performance; our general impression is that it takes longer for these infants to catch on. They are less consistent and are therefore more difficult to manage. They eventually perform as well as the first group of babies, but they take longer and we have to work harder to keep them under experimental control. Finally, about 10 percent of the babies do not meet criterion performance. This may mean that an individual infant discriminated the initial contrast but failed to generalize; it may also mean that the initial contrast was not mastered. Frequently these infants are inattentive and extremely inconsistent with regard to interest in both the visual reinforcer and the toys the assistant uses to hold the infant's attention between trials.

Since we observe infants over a period of about two weeks in almost daily sessions, it is our general impression that these differences among infants are real ones and do not simply represent sampling error. Until follow-up studies are carefully conducted with these groups of infants, or until someone undertakes a comparison study involving presumed normal infants and infants at risk, the application of these techniques to the early identification of infants who will have language difficulties must be considered highly speculative.

In addition, evidence is accruing from a variety of sources that auditory perceptual deficits—for complex acoustic stimuli whether speech or nonspeech —co-occur with language impairment.[66, 67] (See also Tallal, pp 81; Johnston, pp 135; and Sloan, pp 101.) If this is the case, research that is directed towards understanding the characteristics and development of the auditory behavior of infants may eventually provide clues to the further understanding of these deficits, as well as to their early identification. We may also further our knowledge of the relationship between auditory perceptual development and language and speech.

REFERENCES

1. Eimas PD, Siqueland ER, Jusczyk P, Vigorito J: Speech perception in infants. Science 171:303–306, 1971
2. Morse PA: The discrimination of speech and nonspeech stimuli in early infancy. J Exp Child Psychol 14:477–492, 1972
3. Eimas PD: Auditory and linguistic processing of cues for place of articulation by infants. Percept Psychophysiol 16:513–521, 1974
4. Eilers R, Minifie F: Fricative discrimination in early infancy. J Speech Hear Res 18: 158–169, 1975
5. Eimas PD: Auditory and phonetic coding of the cues for speech: Discrimination of the [r-l] distinction by young infants. Percept Psychophysiol 18:341–347, 1975
6. Liberman AM, Delattre PC, Gerstman LJ, Cooper FS: Tempo of frequency change as a cue for distinguishing classes of speech sounds, in Lehiste I (ed): Acoustic Phonetics. Cambridge, M.I.T. Press, 1967
7. Hillenbrand J, Minifie FD, Edwards TJ: Tempo of frequency change as a cue in speech-sound discrimination by infants. J Speech Hear Res 22:147–165, 1979
8. Jusczyk PW: Perception of syllable-final stop consonants by two-month-old infants. Percept Psychophysiol 21:450–454, 1977
9. Jusczyk P, Thompson E: Perception of a phonetic contrast in multisyllabic utterances by two-month-old infants. Percept Psychophysiol 23:105–109, 1978
10. Jusczyk PW, Copan H, Thompson E: Perception by 2-month-old infants of glide contrasts in multisyllabic utterances. Percept Psychophysiol 24:515–520, 1978
11. Trehub S: Infants' sensitivity to vowel and tonal contrasts. Dev Psychol 9:91–96, 1973
12. Swoboda P, Morse P, Leavitt L: Continuous vowel discrimination in normal and at-risk infants. Child Devel 47:459–465, 1976
13. Eilers RE, Wilson WR, Moore JM: Developmental changes in speech discrimination in infants. J Speech Hear Res 20:766–780, 1977
14. Kuhl PK: Predispositions for the perception of speech-sound categories: A species-specific phenomenon? in Minifie FD, Lloyd LL (eds): Communicative and Cognitive Abilities -Early Behavioral Assessment. Baltimore, University Park Press, 1978, 229–255
15. Studdert-Kennedy M, Shankweiler D: Hemispheric specialization for speech perception. J Acoust Soc Am 48:579–594, 1970
16. Liberman AM, Cooper FS, Shankweiler DP, Studdert-Kennedy M: Perception of the speech code. Psychol Rev 74:431–460, 1967
17. Stevens KN, Blumstein SE: Invariant cues for place of articulation in stop consonants. J Acoust Soc Am 64:1358–1368, 1978
18. Blumstein SE, Stevens KN: Acoustic invariance in speech production: Evidence from measurements of the spectral characteristics of stop consonants. J Acoust Soc Am 66:1001–1017, 1979
19. Searle CL, Jacobson Z, Rayment SG: Stop consonant discrimination based on human audition. J Acoust Soc Am 65:799–809, 1979
20. Kuhl PK: Speech perception: Recent approaches, in Lass NJ, Northern JL, Yoder DE, McReynolds LV (eds): Speech, Language and Hearing. Philadelphia, W.B. Saunders, (In Press)
21. Mattingly IG, Liberman AM, Syrdal AK, Halwes T: Discrimination in speech and non-speech modes. Cognitive Psychol 2:131–157, 1971
22. Cutting JE, Rosner BS: Categories and boundaries in speech and music. Percept Psychophysiol 16:546–570, 1974
23. Miller J, Wier C, Pastore R, et al: Discrimination and labeling of noise-buzz sequences with

varying noise-lead times: An example of categorical perception. J Acoust Soc Am 60:410–417, 1976

24. Pastore RE: Categorical perception: A critical re-evaluation, in Hirsh SK, Eldredge DH, Hirsh IJ, Silverman SR (eds): Hearing and Davis: Essays Honoring Hallowell Davis. St. Louis, Washington University Press, 1976, pp 253–264
25. Pisoni DB: Identification and discrimination of the relative onset time of two-consonant tones: Implications for voicing perception in stops. J Acoust Soc Am 61:1352–1361, 1977
26. Carney AE, Widen GP, Viemeister NF: Noncategorical perception of stop consonants differing in VOT. J Acoust Soc Am 62:960--970, 1977
27. Pisoni DB: Auditory and phonetic memory codes in the discrimination of consonants and vowels. Percept Psychophysiol 13:253–260, 1973
28. Pisoni DB, Lazarus JH: Categorical and noncategorical modes of speech perception along the voicing continuum. J Acoust Soc Am 55:328–333, 1974
29. Eimas PD: Linguistic processing of speech by young infants, in Schiefelbusch RL, Lloyd LL (eds): Language Perspectives: Acquisition, Retardation and Intervention. Baltimore, University Park Press, 1974, pp 55–74
30. Morse PA: Infant speech perception: A preliminary model and review of the literature, in Schiefelbucsh RL, Lloyd LL (eds): Language Perspectives: Acquisition, Retardation and Intervention. Baltimore, University Park Press, 1974, pp 19–54
31. Siqueland ER, Delucia CA: Visual reinforcement of non-nutritive sucking in human infants. Science 165:1144–1146, 1969
32. Kuhl PK, Miller JD: Speech perception by the chinchilla: Voiced-voiceless distinction in alveolar plosive consonants. Science 190:69–72, 1975
33. Trehub SE, Chang HW: Speech as reinforcing stimulation for infants. Develop Psychol 6:74–77, 1972
34. Williams L, Golenski J: Infant speech sound discrimination: The effects of contingent versus noncontingent stimulus presentation. Child Develop 49:213–217, 1978
35. Eimas PD: in Cohen LB, Salapatck, P (eds): Speech perception in early infancy, From Sensation to Cognition, vol. I. New York, Academic Press, 1975, pp 193–231
36. Streeter L: Language perception of two-month-old infants shows effects of both innate mechanisms and experience. Nature 259:39–41, 1976
37. Lasky RE, Syrdal-Lasky A, Klein RE: VOT discrimination by four- to six-and-a-half-month-old infants from Spanish environments. J Exp Psychol 20:215–225, 1975
38. Kuhl PK, Miller JM: Speech perception by the chinchilla: Identification for synthetic VOT stimuli. J Acoust Soc Am 63:905–917, 1978
39. Eilers RE, Wilson WR, Moore JM: Speech discrimination in language-innocent and language-wise: A study in the perception of voice onset time. J Child Lang 6:1–18, 1979
40. Eilers R, Gavin W, Wilson W: Linguistic experience and phonetic perception in infancy. Child Devel 50:14–18, 1979
41. Aslin RN, Hennessy B, Pisoni DB, Perez AJ: Individual infant's discrimination of voice onset time: Evidence for three modes of voicing. Paper presented at the Society for Research on Child Development, San Francisco, 1979
42. Gibson EJ: Principles of Perceptual Learning and Development. New York, Appleton-Century-Crofts, 1969
43. Zinchenko VP, van Chzhi-Tsin, Tarakonov VV: The formation and development of perceptual activity. Sov Psychol Psychiatr 2:3–12, 1963
44. Vurpillot E: The development of scanning strategies and their relation to visual differentiation. J Exp Child Psychol 6:622–650, 1968

45. Maccoby EE, Hagen JW: Effects of distraction upon central versus incidental recall: Developmental trends. J Exp Child Psychol 2:280–289, 1965
46. Fodor JA, Garrett MF, Brill SL: Pi ka pu: The perception of speech sounds by pre-linguistic infants. Percept Psychophysiol 18:74–78, 1975
47. Delattre PC, Liberman AM, Cooper FS: Voyelles synthetilues a deux formantes et voyelles cardinales. Maitre Phonetique 96:30–36, 1951
48. Lindblom BEF: Spectrographic study of vowel reduction. J Acoust Soc Am 35:1773–1781, 1963
49. House AS, Fairbanks G: The influence of consonant environment upon the secondary acoustical characteristics of vowels. J Acoust Soc Am 25:105–113, 1953
50. Stevens KN, House AS: Perturbation of vowel articulations by consonantal context: An acoustical study. J Speech Hear Res 6:111–128, 1963
51. Stevens KN, House AS: An acoustical theory of vowel production and some of its implications. J Speech Hear Res 4:303–320, 1961
52. Peterson GE, Barney HL: Control methods used in a study of the vowels. J Acoust Soc Am 24:175–184, 1952
53. Fant G: Acoustic Theory of Speech Production. The Hague, Mouton, 1960
54. Ward WD: Musical perception, in Tobias JV (ed): Foundations of Modern Auditory Theory, Vol 1. New York, Academic Press, 1970, pp 405–554
55. Fant G: Speech Sounds and Features. Cambridge, M.I.T. Press, 1973
56. Joos MA: Acoustic phonetics. Language Supplement 24:1–136, 1948
57. Gerstman LH: Classification of self-normalized vowels. IEEE Trans Audio Electroacoust AU-16:78–80, 1968
58. Lieberman P: On the evolution of language: A unified view. Cognition 2:59–94, 1973
59. Shankweiler D, Strange W, Verbrugge R: Speech and the problem of perceptual constancy, in Shaw R, Bransford J (eds): Perceiving Acting, and Knowing: Toward an Ecological Psychology. New York, Lawrence Erlbaum, 1977, pp 315–346
60. Verbrugge R, Strange W, Shankweiler DP: What information enables a listener to map a talker's vowel space? Haskins Laboratories Status Reports on Speech Research SR-37/38:199–208, 1974
61. Crystal D: Non-segmental phonology in language acquisition: A review of the issues. Lingua 32:1–45, 1973
62. Kuhl PK: Speech perception in early infancy: Perceptual constancy for spectrally dissimilar vowel categories. J Acoust Soc Am 66:1668–1679, 1979
63. Wilson WR, Moore JM, Thompson G: Auditory thresholds of infants utilizing Visual Reinforcement Audiometry (VRA). Paper presented at the American Speech and Hearing Association Convention, Houston, 1976
64. Holmberg TL, Morgan KA, Kuhl PK: Speech perception in early infancy: Discrimination of fricative consonants. J Acoust Soc Am 62 (Suppl 1): S99(A), 1977
65. Kuhl PK, Hillenbrand J: Speech perception in early infancy: Perceptual constancy for categories based on pitch contour. Paper presented at the Society for Research on Child Development, March, 1979
66. Efron R: Temporal perception, aphasia, and déjà vu. Brain 86:403–424, 1963
67. Swisher L, Hirsh IJ: Brain damage and the ordering of two temporally successive stimuli. Neuropsychologia 10:137–152, 1972

Philip J. Levinson and
Marie K. Poulsen*

4

The Development of Sound-Meaning Correspondence During the Sensorimotor Period

The child at the end of the sensorimotor period of intelligence has developed an extensive array of symbolic behaviors. These behaviors, in order of increasing complexity, include deferred imitation, symbolic play, graphic imagery, mental image, and language. These are related in that they suggest a well-developed ability to mentally represent an object or event that is not perceptually present. The focus of this chapter will be on the young child's responses to auditory stimulation during the sensorimotor stage of development and what these responses suggest about the relationship between sound and meaning in the development of language.

Within the framework of Piaget's theory, language is only a particular form of symbolic function that first appears between 18 months and 2 years. Piaget describes this function as the ability to represent something by means of something else which he calls the signifier (sign or symbol) and which is differentiated from that which is signified (object or event). For example, when a toddler picks up a branch and starts sweeping the walk, we know he has the mental image of some object and some prior event. We know the child has the ability to represent the object and the event by means of a signifier (the branch and the sweeping gesture) which is differentiated and not related to the signified (the actual sweeping with a broom). The signifier serves a represen-

---

Preparation of this chapter was supported, in part, by MCH Grant MCT 000914-14-0.
*Authors are listed alphabetically.

tational purpose which allows the child to evoke that which is outside his immediate experience. In following the child's development through the sensorimotor stage, one can observe prelinguistic (presymbolic) behaviors which suggest an orderly progression from an undifferentiated signifier as seen in the signal and index to a differentiated signifier evidenced by the symbol and sign. The signal and index are undifferentiated signifiers. They are concrete attributes of an object or event which serve to set a familiar schema into action. For example, a hanging mobile may serve as a signal to the infant that there is something to reach for, or the opening of a refrigerator may serve as an index that is time to crawl to the high chair for dinner.

Piaget notes that figurative intellectual development* (which would include language) is dependent on four factors:

1. biologic mechanisms available at birth
2. experiences
3. social interaction
4. equilibration.

Consideration of some of the literature provides information regarding the relationship between these factors and aspects of auditory processing. Several studies of infant responses to acoustic information suggest that some abilities are available from birth onward[1-8] while other studies suggest that some abilities are dependent on experience.[6-10]

Eimas[5] in his review of the speech perception literature noted that infants, from birth onward, may perceive speech in the same manner in which adults perceive many speech sounds, a manner approximating categorical perception. He pointed out that this form of perceptual processing suggests an ability to recognize and process speech as speech. This ability has several advantages in terms of language acquisition, specifically sound-meaning correspondence. First, it eliminates the infant's need to learn to differentiate speech as a special class of acoustic signals requiring further analysis to extract the linguistic information. Second, it enables the infant to segment an essentially continuous acoustic input into discrete elements. Finally, it may have an effect on the social bonding between parents and offspring.[4] Mattingly[4] has argued that speech may have functioned early in man's prelinguistic evolutionary history as a sign stimulus for the release of a variety of social behaviors. Such behavior would have helped to establish and maintain the social bonding between infants and their caretakers with the consequence that

*Figurative aspects of intelligence characterize forms of cognition which "from the subjects point of view appear as 'copies' of reality." [p. 653][30] Operative aspects of intelligence characterize forms of cognition which "consist in modifying an object or an event so as to grasp the actual transformations and their results." [p. 654][30]

there would be more opportunity for social interaction, some of which, on the part of the parents, would be linguistic in nature. If speech were still to serve this function, then speech would be one means by which the infant maintains close contact with those who are most likely to provide him with maximum linguistic input and experience.

There is evidence that the discrimination of some speech contrasts is obtainable virtually from birth onward while discrimination of others is more difficult and requires considerable experience. Eilers and Minifie,[6] using a high amplitude sucking paradigm, demonstrated that infants under four months could discriminate among the fricative consonants /sa/ and /va/ and /sa/ and /ʃa/ but could not discriminate between /sa/ and /za/ and /f/ and /ɵ/. Eilers, Wilson and Moore[7] compared the perception of speech contrasts in one- to three-month-old infants, six-to eight-month-old infants, and twelve-to fourteen-month-old infants. Their results indicated that there were contrasts discriminated by all three age groups (/sa/ vs /va/; /sa/ vs /ʃa/); contrasts discriminated by only the two older groups (/sa/ vs /za/; /a:s/ vs /a:z/); and contrasts discriminated by only the oldest group (/fi/ vs /ɵi/).

There is other evidence[9, 10] that suggests that experience affects the manner in which infants respond to auditory stimulation. Anderson[9] compared averaged electroencephalic response (AER) amplitudes in four-month-old infants to: 1. white noise; 2. a two-formant signal; 3. synthesized /da/. Initially all three stimuli evoked noteable responses. After a considerable period of time the stimuli more similar to speech (/da/ and the two-formant signal) produced greater AER amplitudes than the white noise. Anderson explained the results in terms of a learning paradigm. He suggested that complexity (number of features) and pattern (arrangement of features) are key factors affecting the amount of time an infant spends attending to a stimulus. Less complex patterns receive less attention than more complex patterns, although all stimuli receive some attention regardless of how simple and unpatterned. As the stimulus is learned, the response to it is increasingly inhibited until the pattern is learned.

Friedlander[10] investigated responses to complex acoustic stimuli in eleven- to thirteen-month-old infants. In one study, using high-redundancy and low- redundancy messages, he found that initially, subjects spent equal time listening to both sets of messages, then longer to the high-redundancy message, and finally longer to the low-redundancy message. Friedlander suggested that the subjects learned the pattern of the high-redundancy message resulting in a preference for the low-redundancy message. This explanation seems analogous to the one offered by Anderson.[9]

In summary, the literature suggests that there are biologic mechanisms available at birth to process speech as speech and to make certain sound discriminations. It further suggests that[8] experience plays a central role in infant speech perception . . . the specific form of the experience influences the specific form of the perceptual capacities, just how the child makes use of this experience is unclear. At the very least he must be engaged in an active analysis of the frequency of occurrence of speech sounds at various points along phonetic continuum long before these sounds are associated with arbitrary linguistic meanings. [p. 17]

In order to better understand the child's capacity to develop sound-meaning correspondence, it is necessary to view his responses to auditory stimulation within the total framework of symbolic functioning. By observing the child's behaviors, it is possible to trace the evolution of the symbolic function from "sensory/motor assimilation and accommodation* to the mental assimilation and accommodation which characterizes the beginning of representation" [p. 2][11] The forms that these behaviors take are play, imitation, and receptive and expressive language. The development of these behaviors reflects a progression of the symbolic function from the primitive undifferentiated signifiers of the signal and index to the differentiated signifiers of the symbol and sign.

DEVELOPMENT IN THE SENSORIMOTOR PERIOD

Stage I

For the neonate, the need to function is centered in the need for repetition of the inborn behavior patterns of sucking, regarding, listening, vocalizing, and grasping. The exercise of these existing action schemas lead to their adaptation and development as they become progressively differentiated, coordinated, and integrated through experience. According to Piaget,[12] "the reflex is consolidated and strengthened by virtue of its own functioning." [p. 32]

The neonate, through recognitory and generalizing assimilations, develops sensorimotor recognition which enables him to adapt himself to different objects, persons, or auditory events. The first type of signification is the elementary sensory impression accompanying the exercise of the inborn schema and the signified is the schema itself. Generalizing assimilation involves the incorporation of increasingly varied objects or events into the reflex schemas. Recognitory assimilation involves the selectivity which the neonate uses in applying behavioral schemas. For example, the neonate early learns to differentiate his mother's voice.[13] According to Piaget,[11]

the reflex must be conceived as an organized totality whose nature it is to preserve itself by functioning and consequently to function sooner or later for its own sake

*Assimilation is that aspect of intelligence which incorporates reality data by modifying it to fit internal schemes.[12] Accommodation is that aspect of intelligence which modifies internal schemes to fit reality.[25]

(repetition), while incorporating into itself objects propitious to this functioning (generalized assimilation) and discerning situations necessary to certain special modes of its activity (motor recognition). [p. 38]

A characteristic of this stage is the apparent isolation of the inborn schemas of vocalizing, listening, and regarding. The neonate makes no attempt to vocalize to a social, auditory, or visual stimulus. Neither has he developed a system for the visual search of sources of stimulation. The activation of one schema (listening) does not signal attention of another schema (searching).

Imitation is not clearly manifested during Stage I. The neonate will cry in response to other crying infants in the nursery.

At 0; 0 (3) he was drowsy, but not actually asleep, when one of the other babies began to wail; he himself thereupon began to cry. [p. 7]

This may be seen as a contagious or reflexive response to an external stimulus, though Piaget[12] suggests the reflexive notion must be received with caution. Insofar as the reflexive crying response leads to repetition, it sets the stage for the time when the reflexive response will give rise to imitation.

The origin of play is found in the reflexive stage when the neonate exercises inborn action schemas when they do not lead to an adaptive end, for example, sucking schemas activated apart from meals.

Vocalizing is present at birth, and appears to have biologic determinants. The newborn infant cries almost immediately upon waking. Early crying changes in pitch and intensity usually signal bodily discomfort.[14] Differential crying, for example pain vs anger, has been noted by Wolff[15] and Gresell.[16] Intensity and manner of crying may vary with cause and circumstance. The infant's differential cries are signals to mother who then interprets his needs. The interpretation is critical because that is what lends meaning to the cry. Noncrying expressive sounds include small vague throaty noises.[16] Most frequent vowel-like sounds include /ɛ/, /æ/, and /ʌ̂/.[17]

Listening, as an action schema, is also present from birth. The neonate has the capacity to respond selectively to different auditory signals.[5, 18, 19] However, the data suggest that "differential signal recognition in newborns is relatively crude compared to the exquisitely refined acoustical discriminations that become possible later in development." [p. 10][10] When involved in low level motor activity, the neonate will respond to the articulated phones of adult speech with precise synchronized movements.[20] The neonate reacts with global somatic response to nonspeech auditory stimuli; the bell or mother's voice will elicit gross somatic changes or undefined facial responses. The active neonate will become quiet and the quiet baby may become active. The neurologically intact neonate will habituate to continual bell ringing or other loud noises and thus protects himself by being able to turn off an onslaught of aversive stimuli.

Stage II

Stage II is characterized by the transition from inborn to acquired behavior patterns. Some significant habits centering on the infant's own body emerge in the early months. Early vocalizing becomes modified and now differentially signals specific events of pleasure and displeasure.[16, 21] The infant no longer emits sounds by chance, but has learned that his chance sound actions have led to certain results and perceiving these results causes him to repeat the action.[17] Crying itself is prolonged oftentimes because of the interesting sound.[12] According to Wolff,[15] the infant discovers new sounds during precrying fussing and practices them when he is alert and nonfussy. Self-initiated sound play is seen as the infant vocalizes. Cooing sound schemas develop their own primary circular reaction structure in this manner.[11]

During Stage II, the infant begins to respond vocally to auditory and visual stimulation and to the anticipation of events in which he is to be involved (for example, feeding, dressing, being held). The link-up between regarding and vocalizing is noted as the infant spontaneously vocalizes to people and objects. The hook-up is gradual. At first the vocalizations are emitted only to a smiling, touching, talking caretaker.[21] The infant assimilates many such experiences and within weeks spontaneously vocalizes to the presence of a human face.[21]

Mutual imitation begins as the infant continues to produce sounds immediately after his mother imitates him. The sound mechanisms must be in action. The infant is unable to imitate sounds of others unless he is already in the process of making those sounds.[11] It must be noted that the infant does not attempt to approximate the outside sound he hears but rather continues to vocalize his own previously uttered sound. This primitive form of imitation is the foundation for the infant's "gradual expansion of his repertoire of experiences". [p 11][11] Toward the third month, intentional sporadic imitation can be observed. On occasion the infant will imitate a known sound without having uttered it immediately before.[11]

It is during Stage II of sensorimotor development that active listening first becomes apparent. The infant now frequently turns his eyes toward the source of the sound. Isolated behavior patterns fade as coordination among ready-made reflexive schemas begins to emerge. Sounds heard, gradually become something to look at. For example, initially an infant may merely interrupt crying when a sound is heard. Gradually the infant smiles upon hearing the voice, and then begins to search for the source of the sound. In time he becomes adept at systematically locating the source of auditory stimulation.[12, 16, 21] A sound has become a signal to look for its source even when it is not immediately present.

By this time the infant has also learned some basic auditory discriminations as he differentially reacts to the mother's emotional tones. Localization contributes to the infant's ability to make discriminations. Coordinating hearing and vision enables the infant to learn both the visual and auditory characteristics of events, for example, a mother's voice and face vs a stranger's voice and face. In this way, auditory characteristics become concrete attributes of persons or events in the absence of visual input. The coordination of auditory and visual experiences thus contributes to the infant's ability to treat auditory experiences as primitive signifiers.

Primitive signifiers can be either component in the coordination of schemas. For example, a sound may signal a search or an object seen may signal listening. The key notion at this stage is that signifiers are an undifferentiated part of the total organized structure and serve only to release action. The activation of one action component signals activation of the entire structure.

Stage III

Stage III is characterized by the transition from body-centered to object-centered motor activity. Around the fourth month, the infant is no longer confined to activities focused on his own body but becomes interested in the environmental effects of these activities. The primary circular reactions of listening, looking, grasping, and cooing become integrated into secondary circular reactions and are mapped on objects in his environment. The infant acts upon an object with a variety of schemas and then selects that schema which is most effective and reproduces it to continue a particular effect. Interest in sound production emerges as he experiments with shakers, rattles, bells, and other noise making toys.

In this stage, the infant performs an operation of connecting a signal with the schemas related to such activities as feeding, dressing, and socializing. The significations have exclusively a practical meaning; that is, an environmental event becomes a signal to perform an entire action pattern. For example, the squeeze toy becomes a signal for looking, reaching, listening, pulling, and squeezing to produce a sound. The signal entails limited foresight. The signal is not produced by the infant but is only understood by him in a particular context. The signification does not have a representational purpose. It merely sets in motion a certain attitude of expectation and a certain schema of recognition of people and objects.[12]

The first step toward the internalization of action is made as the infant recognizes certain objects or auditory events. For example, he will open his mouth in anticipation of feeding once he has seen the bottle or the spoon. The signified (event) is not differentiated from the signifier (the aspect of the event which provoked the infant's response) and this demonstrates that the approximation to thought is only in its most primitive form. The signals are linked with immediate action and do not give rise to anticipation beyond immediate perception.[11]

A significant cognitive hallmark is made as the infant learns to recognize an object from its parts. The beginning of the index (which emerges in Stage IV) is seen in the primitive signal where a part of the whole can be a signifier of the total object or event for the infant. The barking of a dog signifies the dog as their pet. The creaking of the door signifies mother is about to enter and causes the fussy baby to quiet. The signal is a concrete signifier connected with direct perception and not representation.[12] In general, a signal and even later the index is any sensory impression or directly perceived quality whose signification is an object or sensorimotor schema.[12]

Imitation has advanced from sporadic imitations to systematic intentional imitation. The infant consistently imitates sounds he hears provided they are familiar to him and already a part of his repertoire. The infant thus evidences a discrimination in recognition of sound and movement. This implies he has a memory for the coordination needed to reproduce them.

The infant can respond to words paired with gestures. He will wave to mommy waving while she says 'bye-bye', or claps to mommy clapping while she says, 'pat-a-cake'. This physical imitation paired with a verbal sign sets the stage for the response when mother later will use the verbal signs alone to elicit the waving or clapping response.

Play is seen when action schemas are no longer accompanied by accommodation and therefore, there is no longer any effort at comprehension of the event. When there is merely assimilation to the action itself for the sake of pleasure rather than for comprehension, the infant is indulging in play.

Vocalization and movements are used by the infant to signal for the continuation of activities of caressing, feeding, and playing. The infant is beginning to exercise control of his external environment after discovering his ability to sustain interesting events. The need involved in the act of signaling is the need for repetition. The signal given by the infant sustains rather than initiates an event and thus does not yet constitute a true intelligent act.

The infant vocalizes pleasure and displeasure and gives vocal expression to recognition. His expressive signals are tied to immediate content or context. The sound (signifier) and meaning (signified) in language at this stage appear fused and undifferentiated. The infant has learned to articulate several well-defined syllables. His repetitive babbling of these sounds is essentially for play.

Listening skills continue to emerge. Primitive relations develop in the early months as demonstrated by the infant's ability to discriminate between loud and soft rattle sounds. He can relate sounds and movements demonstrating an understanding that the intensity of his movements is directy related to the intensity of sounds made by the rattle.

The infant begins to listen attentively to the speech of the family and can distinguish friendly and angry talk. He can discriminate specific vowel sounds in his everyday behavior. The infant will selectively listen to familiar words such as 'daddy', 'kitty,' or 'grandma',[21] but does not yet look towards the referent. This suggests these particular sound patterns are familiar to the infant even though symbolic meaning has not been attached to them.

Stage IV

Stage IV is characterized by the emergence of the use of practical intelligence and the index. These aspects of sensorimotor intelligence are critical to the development of symbolic behavior and to the use of language as a tool.

Practical intelligence is seen as goal-oriented behavior. The infant has an objective and tries several known methods to achieve it until he discovers one that works. Actions that are successful are repeated in analogous situations. This goal-directed behavior is both intentional and anticipatory. The methods the infant uses are based on action schemas developed during the preceding stages. These action schemas are generalized, that is, freed from old content, and coordinated in novel ways.[22] The result is new forms or schemas which can be used to achieve goals. In behaving in a goal-directed way, the infant demonstrates knowledge of 'tool use.' For example, using a string or blanket to pull an out of reach toy within reach or vocalizing to get mommy to provide food or drink. This goal-directed behavior initiates rather than sustains an event and thus constitutes an intelligent act. The child sees persons other than himself as sources of action and consequently as tools with which goals can be achieved.

The awareness of the adult as a source of action, the vocalizing schemas laid down in earlier stages, and the child's goal-directed behavior contribute to the use of vocalizing as a communicative tool. The child's repetitive babbling used in Stage III for play purposes now is reorganized into simple sound sequences and intonation patterns more closely approximating the infant's native language. These vocalizations are produced in response to people talking to him and are utilized by the infant to evoke responses in others. The infant's expressive verbal communication begins with nonstandard sounds that accompany his actions, for example, 'ah' (hi) to accompany a wave; 'dat' (pat) to accompany clapping; and 'mm' to accompany eating a cracker.[23] Early words accompany gestures and do not substitute for them. Later in this stage either the word or gesture can serve as an index to elicit the total response.

Between six months and a year, vowels and consonant sounds become articulated in clear syllables. 'Dada' and 'mama' are vocalized in a nonspecific way. The caregiver uses the words 'mama' and 'dada' as symbols to represent the infant's mother and father. The caregiver thereby facilitates the organization of the symbolizing process that is developing in the infant.[23]

Verbal signs are recognized as the infant gives gestural responses to familiar words. He now may point to daddy or doggie when named and shows recognition of 'bye-bye' by waving and 'pat-a-cake' by clapping. He turns to his name and withdraws to 'no, no'.

In play behavior at this stage, objects merely serve as an opportunity for activity. Behavior is not directed in an effort to learn, but is rather a display of known actions.

Genuine imitation begins. The infant can imitate actions he cannot see himself perform such as eyeblinking and sticking out his tongue. He begins to imitate new models provided they are not too different from his own spontaneous action, but he is rarely correct on the first trial. The infant begins to imitate new auditory and visual models though he may need many tentative efforts before he can approximate the model. Initially in imitating speech sounds the infant uses indices or shared features as mediators between the new model and his own familiar behavior.[22]

The index appears during Stage IV. This marks the first separation of the signifier and the signified. Evidence supporting this may be observed in the child's attempts to imitate and his approximations to the model. The Stage III infant was dependent on information from his own monitoring system as a basis for imitating; consequently the infant could only imitate actions of a model when the model produced actions that were part of his repertoire. Using production of articulatory sequences as an example, the Stage III child only knows these productions through his own auditory and tacile-kinesthetic feedback and is not able to use visual information to produce new sounds. Consequently, the visual component of an articulatory production is not seen as a component of the total scheme which defines that production, and the child is not able to utilize that information to imitate the model. The initial attempts to separate the whole into its parts and then use those parts as cues to reproduce the whole are assimilatory in nature. For example, initial attempts at imitating an articulatory sequence that the infant has not just made would involve coordinating the visual input with previously existing behaviors and gradually modifying those behaviors until he had succeeded in imitating the model. The infant's attempts at imitation suggest knowledge of shared features between the model and the infant's own schemas. These shared features are used as mediators in accommodating his own schemas to the new behavior of the model. Piaget provides examples of the infant's coordinating visual input with previously existing behaviors and of the infant's knowledge of shared features.[11]

In the case of T. there was no reaction to movements of the mouth or eyes until about 0;9. At 0;9 (21) however, he looked at me attentively when I opened and closed my mouth (without making a sound) and then said *tata* and *papa* (neither had assigned meaning). Obviously, the reason for this reaction was that he recognized the movement I made when I myself said *papa* (he had imitated the sound on the preceding day) and thus assimilated this movement of my lips to the familiar vocal schema. At 0;9 (29), when I opened my mouth (still without making any sound) T. again said *papa,* but this time in a whisper. He did not, however, imitate any movement related to the tongue, eyes or nose. [p. 40]

At 0;9 (16) the sound *gaga* gave rise to a sustained effort. J said *mama,* then *aha,* then *baba, vava,* and finally *papa*. The sound *pipi* (which had no meaning for her) produced *vv,* then *pp . . . pp* and finally *pff.* When I said *poupou* as at 0;8 (28), J. replied *bvv, abou,* then *bvou, bou,* and finally in a whisper, *pou* and *pou . . . ou* [p. 46]

The index is a primitive signifier that allows the anticipation of the immediate future and the reconstruction of the recent past.[11] It is any sensory impression or directly related perceived quality whose signification is an object or sensorimotor schema. The infant notes shared properties of an event, and he is able to use any portion of the event to foresee the total action. The infant has no mental symbol of the event. The index remains a concrete attribute. For example, mother with a purse is the signifier to mother departing, or a screen is a signifier of a hidden object. The signifier and signified are relatively fused, that is, the occurrence of one depends upon the occurrence of the other and thus the signifier only has presymbolic function.

Stage V

Stage V is characterized by intentional motor exploration of unfamiliar objects and events. The child becomes capable of experimenting in order to discover new properties of objects. The toddler cannot mentally anticipate the results of his motor actions and thus must rely on overt trial and error.

This stage gives rise to the development of the symbol in which an image stands for something it resembles. The symbol initially is primitive and seen only in a very familiar context. The signifier is not truly differentiated in that it exhibits some analogous correspondence with the signified. The use of the symbol emerges as the signifier and signified separate and thus are differentiated. They no longer need to co-occur in time and space. The infant represents a situation by imitating it at a later time. The symbol that is developed refers directly to the knowing of an event because it is "constructed or comprehended as a representation by means of the same scheme of knowing that was operative in constructing the known event in the first place".[24] Symbols are idiosyncratic and are ego-involved signifiers. They are created by the infant as the need arises.

Deferred imitation is the most primitive symbol and evolves from the imitative capacities that begin in early infancy. Imitation as a presymbolic function occurs when the baby imitates a model before him. The toddler watches his mother on the telephone and picks up his own phone and telephones with her, often imitating her intonational patterns. This is presymbolic imitation. When he subsequently performs these actions in the absence of mommy phoning, he has internalized the event and thus can imitate it on a deferred basis.

It is the image which provokes imitation and thus has replaced the need for direct perception of the event for imitation to occur. Piaget notes that[25]

> representation in action is thus liberated from sensorimotor requirements of direct perceptual copy and reaches an intermediary level where action, detached from its context, becomes a differentiated signifer and consequently already constitutes in part a representation in thought. [56]

It is not until the advent of symbolic play and drawing that the transition from representation in action to representation in thought is complete.

What happens is that the toddler watches his mother telephoning and assimilates this event to his own schema while accommodating his schemas to the event. The accommodation becomes visible in part when we see him phoning with his mother. Later in the absence of mother phoning, the child makes the event present by means of the same phoning gesture he used when he was with her. Imitation to the present object (the reality demands of the phone in this case) is the aim. The imitative gesture constitutes the beginning of the differentiated signifier, which implies the beginning of thought, as only thought can connect a real situation with that imitated at a later time. The figurative aspect of this situation is the child's phoning gesture. The operative aspect is the same operative schema by which the child assimilated the original perceptual situation, that is knowing the phone.

Derived from imitative capacities is the toddler's capacity to accommodate to the reality demands of objects encountered in daily living activities. The child's response to these objects gives an indication of his understanding. Typical objects to be presented to the one- to two-year-old include a hat, a mirror, paper, crayons, dolls, shoes, toy cars, a telephone, a cup, a comb, and a saucer. The child who is at the early sensorimotor level of development will respond to objects with indiscriminative handling, mouthing, banging, and throwing schemas. The young toddler (12 to 18 months) responds to objects in a discriminative adultomorphic manner through observing and imitating a model, that is, he pushes a car, hugs the doll, talks on the phone, and scribbles on the paper. He generally responds spontaneously to the reality demands of clothing and feeding utensils (shoe, hat, cup, spoon, and glass).

The older toddler (18 to 24 months) spontaneously responds appropriately to all the familiar objects, in so far as the objects used are perceptually close to the real objects which they are meant to represent. The older toddler no longer needs a model. Based on his knowledge of past visual, auditory, and/or motor experiences, he can respond to the objects in the absence of direct perceptual action. Imitation has become deferred and symbolic.

From twelve to twenty-one months, he confines himself to self-related activities. He may feed himself, put a hat on his own head, talk on the phone, and comb his hair, but he does not apply these schemas to a doll or teddy bear.[11, 26, 27]

Symbolic play is another manifestation of the developing symbolic function. Make-believe or symbolic play is essential for the child's development. Whereas deferred imitation demands the child to accommodate to the external reality of a present object (child matches imitation to the reality demands of the telephone), play allows the child to transform external reality to his own needs (the telephone becomes a drum, fingers and 'rat-a-tat' sounds represent guns). In make-believe play, the child constructs his own signifiers to symbolize an object or event.

Through symbolic play, the child re-lives an event or enacts it symbolically for clarification. Because his verbal language is limited, the child creates his own symbols to express ideas and feelings he cannot put into words. Through play the child creates symbols to express his life experience. Piaget comments:[11]

> . . . systematic observation of a game with dolls immediately shows that the purely maternal attitudes of the child are but a fraction of the whole game. In most cases, indeed, the doll serves only as an opportunity for the child to re-live symbolically her own life in order to assimilate more easily its various aspects as well as to resolve daily conflicts and realize unsatisified desires. We can be sure that all the happenings, pleasant and unpleasant, in the child's life will have repercussions on her dolls. [p. 107]

Piaget[11] classifies symbolic play into several types. Initially, the symbolic schema is primitive in form and the child only puts into action a schema associated with his own behavior. Thus, the toddler will pretend to eat, sleep, and comb his hair but will not ascribe these actions to his teddy bear or doll. He practices these actions symbolically and not in real situations, but the symbol is not yet freed as an instrument to thought.

Schemas still have presymbolic functions since the child merely is applying his usual actions to the normal stimulus of that behavior. There is play in that the schemas are used for pleasure, but there is no symbolism. Early presymbolic play activities center on the exercise of daily living skills outside their direct context.

Expressive language includes the use of verbal signs to signal meaning to others. The child's vocabulary is expanding as he begins to imitate meaningful sounds that are new to him and which are typically words in adult speech. Vocalizations increase in variety of sounds and inflection, until they take on a conversational character so strongly marked that the child seems to be carrying on long meaningful conversations in a foreign language.[16]

First words are uttered in close proximity to the situation to which the child's knowing is attached. The toddlers first words are not symbolic, but are intimately tied to his ongoing actions. He uses words to name persons, animals, objects, and events with which he is actively involved, or uses words in order to express his immediate needs and desires. He does not assign a word to one class of objects, but to a number of similar experiences. For example, a year-old child may say 'dog' for any animal playing outside the window. He may say 'mama' whenever he feels threatened or insecure, 'nana' when he is put down for a nap, or 'again' to ask for more milk or to request that tickling be repeated. Though the child is growing in verbal schemes, he still does not have stable conceptual schemas. Early verbal schemes are midway between a sensorimotor schema (tied to action) and a conceptual schema (tied to an idea).

Listening has developed into understanding the names of many familiar objects, persons, pets, and events. The child has begun to more efficiently associate meaning to the sounds he hears and has learned to respond to simple one-step action commands. He recognizes verbal signs for familiar articles of clothing, toys, foods, and persons.

Stage VI

During Stage VI the child moves from being dependent on direct physical experience for knowing reality to being able to use internalized action schemes in the form of representations and inventions. During Stages IV and V the appearance of a signifier (word or imitation of the model) was dependent on the presence of the signified (object or event referred to by the word or behavior to be imitated); the signifier and the signified were still undifferentiated. In Stage VI the schemes become sufficiently independent of immediate perception to be utilized individually or in novel combinations in the absence of the signified; for example, the child now uses words in the absence of the object or event to which the word refers or imitates behavior in the absence of the model. In effect, the child has internal representations of objects, events, and action schemes and may experiment with or coordinate them without any external adjustments, such as those described in Stage IV. These abilities mark the onset of symbolic behavior.[11]

Imitation becomes more detailed, elaborated, and accurate as the child's operative schema becomes more sophisticated. Whereas the one-year-old may repeatedly lift the phone receiver to his ear, the older child will progressively elaborate by dialing, listening, and talking, and later, by communicating the message to his teddy bear. "Imitation is always a continuation of understanding" [p. 75].[11] The child will only imitiate models to the extent that he understands them.

As the child develops, imitation is no longer dependent on the overt action, and the child becomes capable of internally imitating a series of models in the form of images.[11] According to Piaget, imitation becomes the "instrument for the acquisition of an indefinite number of collective signifiers which in turn give rise to a whole series of socialized representations". [p. 280][11] Assessing the presence and quality of deferred or symbolic imitation in the child helps us to evaluate his understanding of his world. By presenting a child with a variety of objects one can view how he responds to the reality demands.

The transition to preconceptual stage of development and true symbolic play occurs when the child begins to project symbolic schema onto new objects. The child now combs, washes, and feeds his teddy bear. Another form of true symbolic play occurs when the child projects imitative schemas onto new objects. Rather than being limited to his own schemas, the child borrows from other models and he and his dolls begin to 'drive a car,' 'wash the dishes,' 'use the telephone,' and 'rock the baby'. The child's play gains symbolic function when the symbolic schemas are dissociated from their usual activity and are applied to new objects. "The separation of the signifer from the signified which then occurs constitutes symbolism". [p. 123][11]

The development of the ludic symbol in symbolic play is characterized by the identification of one object with another and the identification of the child's own body with that of other people or things. Imitation in play is now not related to the present object but to an absent one. As a ludic symbol, the broom is not to sweep with but to ride. Likewise, the branch becomes a broom, the cup becomes a telephone, the hat is now a purse, and the rock has turned into a dog. The child himself becomes an airplane, a rabbit, or Aunt Molly.

Symbolic play, emerging between three and four years, is elaborate, complex, and episodic. Instead of the fragmented, often repetitious play of the previous type, the child will act out a scene or a series of scenes with real or imaginary beings. The child may wash and iron Raggedy Ann's clothes, bathe and dress her, and then take her to Aunt Sally's house under the elm tree, or he may stack the boxes, count the money, and become Mr. Jones at the supermarket. This is the time when the child may use symbolic play to correct a forbidden reality or neutralize a fear. For example, the child will act out such events as: lighting matches, riding a skateboard, getting a shot, or meeting a snake.

There has been literature from Great Britain concerning the development of play in the young child.[26, 28] Lunzer[26] observed that the degree of organization in the play of two- to six-year-olds was the most significant indicator of play maturity. Lowe[29] studied the development of representational play in 244 children between one and three. Some interesting observations included the following:

12-18 months:	Child responds to objects in terms of self-related activities, for example, uses cup, fork, brush, and comb appropriately, and pushes toy car.
21 months:	Doll-related behavior appears; may place man and objects in car.
24 months:	Doll-related behavior is dominant.
30 months:	Doll-related behavior is central; self-related behavior fades; uses objects to represent absent objects; doll starting to become agent in its own right rather than recipient of child's care.

Verbal schemas are at first idiosyncratic in the sense that they depend on the child's own imitative approximation of what he has heard. Semiwords are intermediate between idiosyncratic imitative symbols and true signs. For example, "mamal" may mean the mailman, the door ringing, noise on the porch, a letter, or a magazine. The first verbal schemas are sensorimotor schemas in the process of becoming concepts. The first verbal signs used by the child change in meaning as the point of view of the child changes. That is 'bow-wow' may refer not only to dogs and similar animals but to anything seen from the location from which the first dog was seen.[11]

As the child develops he sees that the "meanings of words do not constantly change because the classes and relations they denote involve a conceptual definition determined once and for all by the social group". [p. 220][11] Conventional language becomes possible when a sign emerges. A sign differs from a symbol in that it has an arbitrary relation to what it signifies, that is, the sign need bear no resemblance to its referent.

As representative thinking develops, language is used to recall events and to describe events and actions. This is the beginning of words in a symbolic context. They represent an action outside the immediate experiential field. Around two years, the child begins to detach words from external action and begins to use them to report past events. A child returning from the park tells her daddy, "birdie in tree, fly away, all gone." Now the verbal schema is detached from the sensorimotor schema and acquires symbolic function. Piaget comments that "the most characteristic effect of the system of verbal signs on the development of intelligence is certainly that it allows for the transformation of sensorimotor schemas into concepts". [p. 99][11]

The development of language plays an important role in the transition from representational images to true concepts. Language makes possible shared meanings and the social intercourse needed to correct the idiosyncratic concepts of children. The young child does not have the cognitive strategies to develop stable concepts. He cannot focus on more than one aspect of a situation or handle relative differences. His thinking lies midway between the notion of one object and that of a class of objects.

Language ages determined by the size of vocabulary of the child, need close scrutiny to determine how the child is using language. Many reportedly large vocabularies of single words and two-word phrases, under close inspection, represent only the child's expression of present objects, ongoing actions, and immediate needs and desires. Words that are only tied to action represent preverbal schemas that do not yet carry a symbolic function.

ASSESSMENT

In the evaluation of the young child's development of sound-meaning correspondence, one needs to consider not only his responses to auditory stimulation, but all behaviors related to the development of symbolic function.

It is only by viewing the child's auditory behavior within a total symbolic framework that one can determine whether there is a specific auditory disability rather than an overall symbolic delay.

Table 4-1 depicts the behaviors that are critical in evaluating the development of symbolic function.

Table 4-1
Critical Sensorimotor Behaviors in the Development of Symbolic Function

Stage I.

1. Is there a change in the infant's behavior in response to auditory stimulation?
2. Does the infant respond differentially to mother's voice?
3. Does the infant habituate when bombarded with auditory stimulation?
4. Does the infant vocalize?
5. Does the infant grasp objects placed in his hand?
6. Does the infant follow a moving object placed in his line of vision?

Stage II.

1. Does the infant search for or localize sources of auditory stimulation?
2. Does the infant vocalize to persons or objects?
3. Does the infant immediately smile in response to his mother talking?
4. Does the infant smile in response to the examiner talking?
5. Does the infant engage in mutual imitation?
6. Does the infant respond to different emotional tones in mother's voice?
7. Is there a change in the infant's behavior indicating anticipation of familiar events, such as dressing, feeding, being held?
8. Does the infant regard objects placed in his hand?

Stage III.

1. Does the infant respond appropriately to familiar sounds, for example, the dog barking, the door opening?
2. Does the infant listen selectively to familiar words, for example, the names of family members or pets?
3. Does the infant respond to a familiar word accompanied by a gesture?
4. Does the infant imitate sounds he already uses?
5. Does the infant use vocalizations to indicate pleasure or displeasure?
6. Does the infant vocalize to indicate his desire for an activity to continue?
7. Does the infant babble sounds in play?
8. Does the infant vocalize 'mama' and 'dada' nonspecifically?
9. Does the infant manipulate an object to produce an effect, for example, shake a rattle, ring a bell, bang a block?
10. Does the infant imitate movements he can see himself doing, for example, clapping his hands, ringing a bell?
11. Does the infant retrieve a partially hidden object?

Stage IV.

1. Does the infant attempt to imitate sounds not in his repertoire?
2. Does the infant use nonstandard sounds to accompany his action?
3. Does the infant vocalize 'mama' and 'dada' to refer to mommy and daddy?
4. Does the infant respond appropriately to familiar words, for example, his name, 'no-no,' 'bye-bye,' and 'pat-a-cake'?
5. Does the infant attempt to imitate facial actions he cannot see himself doing?
6. Does the infant attempt to imitate object to object actions, for example, cube in cup, pencil mark on paper?
7. Does the infant's behavior indicate he anticipates a total event from experiencing a part of the event, for example, key, purse, or coat indicates mother's departure?
8. Does the infant's behavior indicate that he has a particular goal in mind prior to action, for example, crawls around chair to retrieve toy?

Stage V.

1. Does the toddler imitate sounds, words and actions which he has not previously produced?
2. Does the toddler use words to name or request present objects, persons, and events?
3. Does the toddler's "babbling" sound like he's speaking in short sentences?
4. Does the toddler follow one-step directions when accompanied by gestures?
5. Does the toddler indicate that he understands the names of familiar food, clothing, and people?
6. Does the toddler use trial and error to problem solve, for example, dumping a pellet from a bottle?
7. Does the toddler use familiar self-related objects appropriately?
8. Does the toddler use pretend play in self-related actions, for example, in sleeping, eating, and dressing?

Stage VI.

1. Does the toddler spontaneously imitate words and phrases on a deferred basis?
2. Does the toddler talk about objects and events which are not present?
3. Does the toddler combine words into short phrases?
4. Does the toddler follow simple commands without gesture?
5. Does the toddler indicate he understands the names of toys, household objects, and body parts?
6. Does the toddler problem solve without overt trial and error, for example, pushes chair to table to reach a desired object?
7. Does the toddler use household objects appropriately, for example, a broom, a vacuum cleaner, lipstick?
8. Does the toddler pretend play with dolls, for example, feeding, bathing, or dressing a doll or a teddy bear?
9. Does the toddler use pretend play in adult-related actions, for example, driving a car?
10. Does the toddler pretend with objects, for example, uses the broom as a horse or the block as a car?

REFERENCES

1. Moffit AR: Consonant cue perception by twenty to twenty-four-week-old infants. Child Dev 42:717–731, 1971
2. Eimas PD, Siqueland ER, Jusczyk P, Vigorito J: Speech perception in infants. Science 171:303–306, 1971
3. Trehub SE, Robinovitch MS: Auditory-linguistic sensitivity in early infancy. Dev Psychol 6:74–77, 1972
4. Mattingly IG: Speech cues and sign stimuli. Am Sci 60:327–337, 1972
5. Eimas P: Speech perception in early infancy, in Cohen LB, Salapatek P (eds): Infant Perception: From Sensation to Cognition, Vol. 2 Perception of Space, Speech, and Sound. New York, Academic Press, 1975, pp 193–231
6. Eilers RE, Minifie F: Fricative discrimination in early infancy. J Speech Hear Res 18: 158–167, 1975
7. Eilers RE, Wilson WR, Moore JM: Developmental changes in speech discrimination in infants. J Speech Hear Res 20:766–780, 1977
8. Eilers RE, Gavin W, Wilson W: Linguistic experience and phonemic perception in infancy: A cross linguistic study. Child Dev 50:14–18, 1979
9. Anderson D: Averaged electroencephalic responses of infants to speech related stimuli. Unpublished doctoral dissertation, University of Washington, 1973
10. Friedlander BZ: Receptive language development in infancy: Issues and problems, Merrill-Palmer 16:7–51, 1970
11. Piaget J: Play, Dreams, and Imitation in Childhood. New York, W.W. Norton, 1962
12. Piaget J: The Origins of Intelligence in Children. New York, International Universities Press, 1952
13. Babies are people. NOVA, Education in Oregon, PBS, 1979
14. Berry MF, Eisenson J: Speech Disorders: Principles and Practices of Therapy. New York, Appleton-Century-Crofts, 1956

15. Wolff P: The natural history of crying and other vocalizations in early infancy, in Foss BM (ed): Determinants of Infant Behavior IV. London, Metheun and Company, 1969
16. Knobloch H, Pasamanick B (eds): Gesell and Amatruda's Developmental Diagnosis (3rd ed.). New York, Harper and Row, 1974
17. Berry MF: Language Disorders in Children: The Bases and Diagnoses. New York, Appleton-Century-Crofts, 1969
18. Butterfield EC: An extended version of modification of sucking with auditory feedback. Working Paper No. 43, Bureau of Child Research, Children's Rehabilitation Unit, University of Kansas Medical Center, 1968
19. Eisenberg R, Griffin EJ, Coursin DB, Hunter MH: Auditory behavior in the human neonate: A preliminary report. J Speech Hear Res 7:245–269, 1964
20. Condon WS, Sander LW: Synchrony demonstrated between movements of the neonate and adult speech. Child Dev 45:456–462, 1974
21. Bayley N: Bayley Scales of Infant Development. New York, Psychological Corp, 1969
22. Morehead D, Morehead A: From signal to sign: A Piagetian view of thought and language during the first two years, in Schiefelbusch RL, Lloyd LL (eds): Language Perspectives—Acquisition, Retardation, and Intervention. Baltimore, University Park Press, 1974
23. Greenfield PM, Smith JH: The Structure of Communication in Early Language Development. New York, Academic Press, 1976
24. Furth H: Piaget and Knowledge: Theoretical Foundations. Englewood Cliffs, Prentice-Hall, 1969
25. Piaget J, Inhelder B: The Psychology of the Child. New York, Basic Books, 1969
26. Lunzer E: Intellectual development in the play of young children. Educ Rev 11:205–217, 1959
27. Laine M: Trends in the development of representational play in infants from one to three. J Child Psychol Psychiatr 16:33–47, 1975
28. Hulme I, Lunzer E: Play, language, and reasoning in subnormal children. J Child Psychol Psychiatr 7:107–123, 1966
29. Lowe M: Trends in the development of representational play in infants from one to three years: An observational study. J Child Psychol Psychiatr 16:33–47, 1975
30. Oléron P, Piaget J, Inhelder B, Gréco P: Mental images, in Gruber HE, Voneche JJ (eds): The Essential Piaget: An Interpretive Reference and Guide. New York, Basic Books, 1977

Paula Tallal

5
Auditory Processing Disorders in Children

There is no doubt among those working with children with specific developmental language disabilities that these patients have difficulty with various aspects of higher linguistic processing. Evidence for syntactic, semantic, and conceptual deviations among children with language disorders is not difficult to document. However, the results of studies that investigate higher level linguistic and cognitive abilities of children with language disorders can be extremely difficult to interpret. In such children, deviations in linguistic performance might be attributable to difficulty with higher order concepts, syntactic or phonologic rules. However, it is also possible that linguistic or cognitive deficits could result from more primary perceptual problems, for example, a difficulty in detecting multiple signals, in discriminating temporal or spectral features, or in integrating different aspects of complex stimuli over time. Until we can effectively rule out any malfunctions in these more primary perceptual mechanisms, it will be extremely difficult to differentiate between disorders which may arise in the different stages of language processing. If eventually we are to understand the precise etiology of language disorders, and hence to improve diagnosis and therapeutic techniques for dealing with them, it is imperative to investigate in detail, and in a systematic manner, the

*Portions of this chapter have appeared in Tallal, P. Auditory processing disorders in children. *Audio Journal* L. Bradford (ed). New York: Grune and Stratton, 1978, and are reprinted here with permission.

underlying sensory and perceptual hierarchies involved in language, before placing the blame, as it were, on the malfunctioning of higher order linguistic systems.

Most likely, there are important differences between the organization and functions of the developing brain and those of the adult brain. The mechanisms that are required in developing a function and those involved in maintaining that function, once developed, may not be identical. Different mechanisms may be involved in developing a function than are involved in maintaining that function once it has been fully developed. Thus, the effect of hearing impairment on language comprehension may be quite different in the child who has not yet developed language than in the adult who has had many years of successful language experience. In other words, even though the *cause* of the resulting language disability (elevated sensory threshold) may be the same for both the child and the adult, the *effect* of such a loss and the methods needed for remediation might be quite different. Adequate reception of the physical acoustic aspects of the speech signal is an important component to language comprehension for the patient who has become hearing impaired as an adult, but it is not as critical for that person as it is for the child developing language.

Broadbent pointed out that the speech signal is so redundant that if the listener has some knowledge of what to expect, even if only a small part of the signal is intact, its meaning can be adequately derived.[1] However, for the child who has not yet developed knowledge of the structure of language, adequate reception of the physical acoustic aspects of the speech signal is critical. One need only observe the enormous difficulties experienced by most congenitally deaf children attempting to learn language in the absence of normal acoustic input to understand the magnitude of importance of the preliminary auditory analysis stage of speech perception. Blesser has suggested that the problem with deaf children is that their concept of the gross structure of language is not very secure and, therefore, their ability to benefit from redundancies and those other aspects of the acoustic message that are available to them is not adequate.[2]

On the other hand, the same degree of hearing loss that may result in a profound language disorder in the developing child, will not necessarily disrupt expressive language when occurring for the first time in adult life. Similarly, a deficit that affects phonetic analysis may not significantly affect reading ability when it occurs in otherwise normal adults. Nonetheless, the same deficit may result in considerable difficulty in children originally learning how to read. This may be particularly important when a phonics approach to reading is being taught.

As is the case for reading, acoustic and/or phonetic analysis is likely to play a different role in language comprehension in childhood and adulthood.

In order for us to understand this interaction, it is important that developmental studies be done that will investigate which precise mechanisms are involved in speech perception and, subsequently, language development. This approach will, hopefully, elucidate the role of auditory perception in language development and disorders.

It is obvious from observing deaf children that dysfunction in the sensory registration of the auditory signal is sufficient to disrupt speech perception and give rise to a global language disorder. Is there experimental evidence for any other defective sensory or perceptual mechanisms that might underlie other types of communicative disorders?

The role of auditory perception in language disabilities has been an area of controversy for many years. There is mounting evidence now that some patients with language disabilities have specific auditory processing impairments that might underlie their language dysfunction. Knowing, as we do, the devastating effects of impairment of auditory *sensation* on the subsequent language development of hearing impaired children, it seems imperative that we take seriously the mounting evidence of auditory *perceptual* impairments in children with language disabilities.

BACKGROUND LITERATURE PERTAINING TO AUDITORY PROCESSING DISORDERS IN CHILDREN

Ewing demonstrated as early as 1930 that six of ten developmental aphasic children that he studied had raised thresholds for some high frequencies.[3] There is a concensus of opinion now that, with the improvement of audiometric techniques, the kind of hearing loss identified by Ewing can be excluded before arriving at a diagnosis of specific language disability. At the least, it may be said that the degree of simple peripheral hearing loss of this kind in aphasic children is small, if present at all, and not sufficient to explain their severe language retardation.

Other sensory deficits have been reported in children with language problems. Rosenthal and Wohlert reported that developmental aphasic children demonstrated abnormal auditory temporal summation thresholds and masking level differences.[4] However, these and other authors who report the results of psychoacoustic studies that use pure tones or other simple nonverbal acoustic stimuli, have not been able to relate these acoustic deficits to language processing abilities. It is known that certain nonverbal and verbal acoustic processing are substantially different and occur, at least in part, in different hemispheres of the brain. Milner[5] has reviewed this literature. Furthermore, studies by Danaher and Pickett with hearing impaired subjects indicate that sensory deficits alone are not adequate predictors of language disabilities.[6]

If we intend to investigate whether impaired auditory mechanisms are causal in language delay, it is essential that we examine in detail higher level auditory perceptual processes that may be directly involved with speech perception. Clinical descriptions of children with specific developmental language dysfunction have repeatedly suggested that these children have auditory perceptual deficits. In his original definition of the syndrome "Developmental Aphasia", Benton reported that there was evidence suggesting that the basis of the disorder is a high level deficit of auditory perception.[7] Earlier, Monsees stressed the possible importance of temporal sequencing deficits in developmental aphasic children.[8] Hardy also described the aphasic child's difficulties with what he called "auding," the integrative functions in the brain's management of auditory information.[9] He suggested that such difficulties may underlie inability of these children to distinguish between similar sounding words. Eisenson[10, 11, 12] discussed the types of perceptual impairments that have been observed in most aphasic children. These included (1) defective capacity for storing speech signals; (2) impairment of phoneme recognition specifically within contextual utterances; and (3) impairment in processing sequences of speech events at the normal rate at which they occur. These clinical observations have provided a basis for the experimental investigation of the perceptual abilities of dysphasic children. In particular, interest has focused on the role of auditory sequencing and auditory memory.

Lowe and Campbell studied children which they classified as "aphasoid".[13] They used similar methods to those originally employed by Efron[14] in his study of the perception of temporal order in adult aphasic patients. In Lowe and Campbell's experiment, aphasoid children were compared with normal children, matched for age on their ability to judge succession. The term succession here corresponds to Hirsh's[15, 16] definition of auditory fusion, the inter-sound-interval, ISI, at which two stimuli are heard as two sounds rather than one. These children were also tested on their ability to judge temporal order. Two different 15 msec pure tones of 400 Hz and 2200 Hz were presented in rapid sequence with brief ISIs. Subjects were required to indicate which of the two tones occurred first. The results of the study showed that there were no significant differences between the two group's performances on the succession task.[13] In a recent study, Kornet, Thal, and Maxon reported replicating the finding that language delayed children had normal temporal resolution abilities.[17] However, the aphasoid children, compared to the controls, were significantly impaired in their ability to indicate which of two tones occurred first when the tones were presented in rapid succession. The normal controls made correct temporal order judgements at ISIs of from 15 msec to 80 msec. The mean ISI for the group was 35.8 msec. The aphasoid children required intervals of 55 msec to 700 msec, with a mean of 357 msec to achieve the same level of performance as the controls. Lowe and Campbell concluded that disturbed temporal ordering might be a major factor in the communication difficulties of aphasoid children.[13]

Aten and Davis[18] carried out an extensive study of the perception of verbal and nonverbal auditory sequences in children whom they classified as having "minimal cerebral dysfunction" (MCD). Children with one or more definite signs of central nervous system disorder were included in their MCD group. For these authors, evidence of central nervous system disorder included abnormal electroencephalogram, seizures, head injuries, and bilateral hematomas. Tests of nonverbal auditory perception included (1) reproducing rhythmically presented sequences of pure tones, and (2) judging the duration of pure tone sound bursts by selecting a short, medium, or long plastic block corresponding in length to the relative duration of the tone. Tests of verbal perception included (1) serial memory span for nonsense syllables, digits and words, and (2) verbal reproduction of multisyllabic words, scrambled sentences, and paragraphs presented sequentially. The results indicated that, in general, the MCD group performed more poorly than the control group on perceptual memory span and the number of stimuli accurately reproduced. The MCD group was specifically imparied in their ability to respond correctly to auditory stimuli which varied in rhythm and duration. This evidence suggested that perception, storage, and reproduction of sequential auditory stimuli might be disturbed by cerebral dysfunction.

Griffiths[19] reported a study in which developmental aphasic children and normal children were tested for their ability to reproduce nonverbal rhythmic patterns. Rhythmic patterns were tapped in 4/4, 6/8, and 3/4 time on a tambourine at the rate of approximately two quarter notes per second. The subjects were required to reproduce the pattern on another tambourine immediately after they heard it. The aphasic children performed as well as the control subjects on the simplest patterns. This demonstrated that they understood the task and were willing to respond. However, they were markedly impaired in their ability to reproduce the more complex rhythmic patterns that were presented. Griffiths suggests that difficulties in temporal ordering of auditory stimuli, discrimination of relative duration, or reduced memory span could be responsible for the impaired performance of the developmental aphasic children on this task.[19]

Monsees[20] studied the ability of children with expressive language disorders and normal control children to repeat isolated phonemes. Phonemes were presented over a loud speaker in order to eliminate visual cues. The children's ability to make same-different judgements on pairs of nonsense syllables from the *Templin Sound Discrimination Test* was investigated along with their ability to blend a sequence of phonemes into a word, for example, /p/ + /ai/ (pronounced eye) equals "pie". She also studied these children's ability to repeat a sequence of phonemes maintaining the order of their presentation. The results of these experiments showed no significant differences between the abilities of the normal children and the children with expressive language disorders in imitating isolated phonemes. However, the performance of the langauge-impaired group was significantly impaired (in comparison to that of the controls) on all other tasks studied. This study provided evidence that inability of dysphasic and other language impaired children to report the temporal order of nonverbal auditory stimuli, reported in earlier investigations, applied to their performance with verbal stimuli as well.

Rosenthal and Eisenson[21] reported the results of studies comparing aphasic and normal children in their abilities to resolve the temporal order of sounds that differ from one another in acoustic features, particularly those emphasizing speech versus nonspeech characteristics. They required subjects to indicate which member of a pair of auditory stimuli occurred first when the order of stimulus presentation varied randomly. Six stimulus pairs were studied: pure tone-noise pairs (T,N); high tone-low tone pairs (T_1T_2); vowel /a/-affricative pairs (V.A.); vowel /a/-vowel /i/ pairs (V_1V_2); fricative /s-fricative /sh/ pairs (F_1F_2); and fricative /sh/-affricate /ch/ pairs (F_2A). These stimuli were selected in order to contrast certain acoustic features, such as speech vs nonspeech, and frequency information vs temporal information. Natural speech signals were used as stimuli in this experiment.

The results of these studies indicated that the aphasic group was impaired on all tasks studied when compared to the normal subjects. However, this difference in performance was not associated with simple speech vs nonspeech dimensions alone. Both the easiest (V.A.) and most difficult (F_2A) pairs consisted of speech stimuli. Whereas the dysphasic subjects were able to report the order of presentation of V.A. pairs with ISIs of only 64 msec, they required 650 msec to perform to the same level of accuracy with F_2A pairs. In contrast to normal subjects, the dysphasics had greater difficulty in ordering pairs whose members could be differentiated only by analyzing temporally coded features, than in ordering those that could be distinguished by frequency cues. Rosenthal and Eisenson concluded that the nature of the auditory disorder of dysphasic children could be characterized as an inefficiency in auditory temporal analysis.[21]

Poppen and his colleagues[11] have pointed out that several authors report that there are not only auditory perceptual impairments in developmental dysphasic children, but also visual, perceptual, and memory impairments. In Poppen's study of this claim, the sequencing abilities of aphasic, deaf, and normal children were investigated and compared in both visual and auditory modalities. It was found that there were no differences between the aphasic and deaf children, but both of these groups were inferior to normal control children on tasks requiring them to reproduce temporal and spatial sequences of visual stimuli. This suggested that aphasic children exhibit impairments in both the auditory and the visual modality on sequencing tests.[11] It should be emphasized that this conclusion can only be tentative. The visual and auditory stimuli used for comparison in these sequencing tests were not presented in the same manner, that is, either both spatially or both temporally. Since this was the case in these experiments, a direct comparison of modalities cannot be made because of the interacting factors related to stimulus orientation methods.

Other experiments investigating the perceptual abilities of language impaired children have suggested that these children may have both auditory and visual sequencing deficits. However, these studies have been few in number, have utilized quite different criteria for inclusion of subjects into the various experimental groups studied, and have employed different experimental procedures.

An important methodologic difficulty common to all of the experiments investigating sequencing and memory that have been discussed so far, has been the failure to show that subjects were able to discriminate accurately between stimulus elements that were combined and presented in sequence. In every experiment reported, it has been assumed that because discrimination between stimulus elements presented in isolation was demonstrated, deficits in perception of sequences composed of these elements must result from a failure to perceive or remember temporal order. As early as 1959 Hirsh pointed out that in order to perceive the sequence of a two-element stimulus pair, one must first perceive that the two elements are separate rather than fused, and then decide whether they are the same or different.[16] Nevertheless, in the experiments reviewed here that were designed specifically to assess sequencing and memory abilities of language delayed children, no steps were taken to show that subjects could perform these more primary perceptual tasks. Thus, it is possible that the subjects' failure was due to difficulty in discrimination between the two stimuli presented sequentially, even though the subjects had no difficulty discriminating between the stimuli when they were presented singly. If this were the case, then poor performance on tests of perception of temporal order could be attributed to difficulty in discriminating between the items of a stimulus pair, rather than in determining their temporal order. This could well be the case for any experiments investigating the perception of temporal order in language impaired children because they failed to control for accuracy of discrimination of sequentially presented stimuli.

Rees[22] reviewed all of the literature to date on auditory perceptual deficits in language impaired subjects. She criticized these experiments with language impaired subjects on several grounds, emphasizing three particular problems which resulted in difficulties in interpretation:

1. Theories that are based on the results of studies in which pure tones have been used as stimuli can be criticized on the grounds that pure tones could be processed differently from speech sounds.

2. The results of studies that use verbal stimuli to assess the perceptual abilities of language disordered subjects may be confounded by the effects of linguistic ability. In other words, impairment observed in such studies may possibly result from the fact that language delayed children have specific difficulty with verbal stimuli that do not derive from more basic perceptual impairment.
3. Investigators have failed to establish a positive correlation between the extent of perceptual disorder in language impaired subjects and the extent of their associated language impairment.

Rees concluded that even if a primary perceptual difficulty could be isolated in language delayed children, this would not constitute evidence that such problems were systematically related to the language disabilities of these children.

RECENT RESEARCH PERTAINING TO AUDITORY PROCESSING DISORDERS IN CHILDREN

In order to understand the relationship between basic perceptual disorders and language delay, it seemed to be necessary to move away from the previously used experimental procedures and to reevaluate the experimental questions. A new experimental method and new stimuli seemed to be required. A means of generating nonverbal stimuli that imitated the acoustic properties of speech sounds but did not match the acoustic spectrum of any specific phoneme was needed. Such signals could be acoustically speech-like, but at the same time, linguistically meaningless. Recent work in the field of psychoacoustics, together with the development of speech synthesizers, has made it possible to specify and control the critical acoustic features necessary for such signals.

In order to understand the perceptual deficits of children with language delay, it was essential to devise a method which would enable the children to report in detail exactly what they perceived in each stimulus presentation in a nonverbal manner. Furthermore, it was important that the method should be easy to demonstrate without the need for verbal instruction or verbal response. The method also needed to be flexible enough to allow for several different aspects of perception to be investigated systematically by changing only one variable at a time.

It was also important to assure that the results obtained in perceptual studies using nonverbal complex acoustic stimuli could be compared directly to the results of similar studies using nonverbal visual stimuli or verbal stimuli. Furthermore, studies of the relationship between these perceptual abilities and other abilities such as language comprehension and speech production were needed.

In 1970 the author began to work on these issues, initially with Malcolm Piercy in Cambridge, and later with other colleagues including Freda Newcombe in Oxford, England, and Rachel Stark at the Kennedy Institute in Baltimore. In all of our experiments, which will be discussed below, a nonverbal operantly conditioned method was used. This method was designated the Repetition Method.[23]

Method. At the very outset of designing a test of auditory perception, there are some very basic but extremely important principles that must be taken into account. Since auditory perception is an integral part of speech perception, it is clearly important to establish that the results obtained from auditory perceptual tests are not significantly affected by the subjects' ability to understand the test instructions or by his capacity to produce a verbal response. Thus, when designing a perceptual test battery it is essential to eliminate the need for verbal instructions or verbal responses. Another important feature of a perceptual test design should be its flexibility and versatility. The method should allow the subject to report in detail exactly what he has perceived in each stimulus presented, in a nonverbal manner. It should also be flexible enough to allow for several different aspects of perception to be investigated in a hierarchical manner, systematically moving from one subtest to another. The subtests should be arranged in such a way as to begin with the most basic functions of interest and, by changing only a single variable at a time, proceed to more complex functions. Furthermore, the same method should be adaptable to a variety of stimulus materials and should be appropriate for testing in several different sensory modalities.

Stimuli. When selecting stimuli to be used in a test, many of the same issues that apply to designing the test method pertain. As auditory perception is so intimately interrelated with speech perception, the use of verbal stimuli in an auditory perceptual test will lead to confounded results unless careful controls are included. If verbal stimuli are to be included in the test, then it is necessary either to use nonverbal stimuli as well, so that a direct comparison can be made between the two, or to use the test only as a measure of speech perception, rather than auditory perception. This issue is particularly important when the test will be used with patients with known or suspected language disabilities. If verbal stimuli alone are used as test items, then the results of the test can yield information only about speech perception. It will not be possible with such a test to acquire information specifically about auditory perception, because it is possible that these same patients might have responded quite differently had nonverbal stimuli been used. Thus, if we think back to the earlier example of the digit span test, it becomes clear that such a test should not be used, although it often is, as a measure of auditory sequential memory. It is quite possible that auditory sequential memory ability could be intact and yet language ability be such as to interfere with adequate performance on this task. This is a basic criticism of many of the auditory perceptual tests that are presently available for clinical use. That is, they do not measure auditory perception, *per se*.

Another issue of concern when choosing stimuli for an auditory perceptual test is to control, as precisely as possible, the stimulus parameters. For example, if the test is intended to measure auditory sequencing ability, performance on the test may be affected by temporal, spectral, or amplitude differences between the stimuli to be sequenced or the rate of presentation of the stimuli. Changing any of these properties of the stimuli might result in significant changes in the sequencing performance purportedly being measured.

THE REPETITION TEST

Our own work has been directed towards establishing a better understanding of the perceptual prerequisites for normal language development. We have, therefore, been specifically interested in developing new methods for assessing a variety of perceptual abilities of young children with and without delayed language development. In this pursuit, we have attempted to incorporate the concepts discussed in the previous section into a perceptual test battery. The resulting test has come to be known as the Repetition Test. As the test design is such a fundamental aspect of our experimental findings, this will be discussed in detail. Once the method is understood, the results of our perceptual experiments with various subject populations become more meaningful.

In the Repetition Test two different stimuli are used in combination. Subjects are trained, with operant conditioning techniques, to respond to these stimuli by pressing either one or the other of the two identical panels mounted side-by-side on a response box. This method was devised to enable the subject to nonverbally repeat, in detail, exactly what he perceives in each stimulus presentation by making the appropriate motor response. It is important that the two stimulus items can be incorporated into the test method. The test can be given repeatedly with various stimulus pairs as long as the order of presentations of the various stimulus pairs is counter balanced to control for learning or fatigue. The same test procedure can be used to test nonverbal and verbal perception in any sensory modality. Therefore, results obtained using nonverbal acoustic stimuli can be compared directly to those using nonverbal visual or tactile stimuli in order to test for modality differences in the same subject or group of subjects. Similarly, nonverbal perception can be compared directly to verbal perception using this method. Finally, by carefully selecting stimulus pairs to be used in the test, specific aspects of acoustic and phonetic processing can be investigated.

The Repetition Test is made up of a series of subtests. The subtests, described below, are arranged in such a way as to investigate a hierarchical series of perceptual abilities. The subtests must always be given in the following order as each subsequent subtest relies on skills learned in the previous subtest.

Detection. Stimulus 1 is presented and the experimenter shows the subject that the bottom panel on the response box is to be pressed each time stimulus 1 occurs. Stimulus 1 is presented repeatedly until the subject has pressed the bottom panel in response to stimulus 1 ten times in succession. Next, stimulus 2 is presented and the experimenter indicates that the top panel of the response box is to be pressed each time stimulus 2 occurs. Stimulus 2 is presented repeatedly until the subject has pressed the top panel of the response box ten times in succession. Correct performance on this test indicates that the subject can detect the presence of the stimulus and make the correct motor response.

Association. Stimulus 1 or stimulus 2 is presented individually in random order. The subject is trained to respond to each of these stimuli by pushing the appropriate panel on the response box. Training continues until either criterion is reached (20 correct responses out of 24 consecutive presentations) or 48 trials have been given. Correct performance on this subtest indicates that a subject perceives the difference between stimulus 1 and stimulus 2 when each is presented individually, and that he is able to learn to associate each of these stimuli with the correct panel on the response box.

Sequencing Training. In this subtest, for the first time, two stimuli are presented sequentially. Subjects who reach criterion on the association task are trained to respond to each of the four possible two-element sequence patterns (1-1, 1-2, 2-2, 2-1) with a 428 msec inter-sound-interval (ISI) by pushing the panels in the corresponding order. Correct responses are demonstrated for four trials by the experimenter, followed by eight training trials in which knowledge of the results is given to the subject. Next, 24 two-element patterns are presented randomly; the subject receives no information about the results. For subjects who reach criterion on this task, it can be determined that they are able to detect that two stimuli were presented, to determine whether they were the same two stimuli or two different ones and, if they were two different ones, to indicate the order in which they occurred. For subjects who do not reach criterion on this subtest (make more than 14 errors) two additional subtests are given to determine at what point the difficulty arose. That is, did their difficulty result from an inability to perceive that two signals were presented, to discriminate between the two signals, or to perceive their temporal order?

Same/Not Same. Subjects who failed to reach criterion on sequencing training are tested further. The same two-element patterns that were presented in sequencing training are presented again in this subtest. The response box is turned by 90 ° to avoid confusion between the two tasks. The subject is initially presented with two identical stimuli, separated by a 428 msec ISI, and trained to press the right panel to indicate that the two stimuli are the same as each other. Then the subject is presented with two different stimuli, separated by a 428 msec ISI, and trained to press the left panel to indicate that the two stimuli are not the same as each other. Visual examples are used in training to assure that all subjects fully understand the response required on this task. Then, the subject is presented with the same series of two-element sequences that were used in the sequencing training subtest. However, in this case, the subject is required only to respond to whether the two elements in the sequence are the same or not the same as each other. If, after 48 trials a subject fails to reach the criterion, he is not continued further on this test using the same stimulus items. Once the subject reaches the criterion, the same series of 24 two-element patterns with ISIs between 8 and 305 msec that are used in the sequencing test with short ISIs (described below) are presented. However, this time the subject will be required only to indicate whether the two stimuli in each sequenced pattern were the same or not the same as each other.

It is important to note that the same stimli are given in the sequencing and the same/not same subtest. In the sequencing subtest, knowledge of the order of the stimuli is required; in the same/not same subtest, knowledge of temporal order is not required. If a subject failed to reach criterion on the sequencing subtest, but did reach criterion on the same/not same subtest, then this subject is having difficulty in perceiving the temporal order in which the stimuli are presented. However, if a subject failed to reach criterion on both the sequencing and the same/not same subtest, then this subject is having difficulty perceiving the sound quality of the two stimuli, that is, he cannot discriminate between them. If the subject cannot discriminate between two stimuli, he will also not be able to sequence them. It would be incorrect to say that this subject had difficulty in sequencing. His sequencing ability may be adequate once the stimuli to be sequenced can be discriminated.

Sequencing with Short ISIs. Subjects who reach criterion on the sequencing training subtests are tested further. The same series of 24 two-element stimulus patterns that were used in the sequencing training subtest are presented again. However, in this subtest, the duration of the interval between the offset of the first element and the onset of the second element in the stimulus pattern, the ISI, is varied. ISIs of 8, 15, 30, 60, 150, and 305 msec are presented randomly, four trials at each ISI. Subjects who reached criterion on the sequencing training subtest, but who have difficulty with this subtest, fail because of the rapid rate of presentation of the stimulus items.

Sequencing with Long ISIs. The same series of 24 two-element stimulus patterns used above are presented again. In this subtest the duration of the ISI is varied between 947 and 4062 msec (947, 1466, 1985, 3023, 3543, and 4062 msec); four trials at each ISI are presented randomly. The subject is trained to wait until both elements in the stimulus pattern have been presented before responding. This places additional demands on short-term memory. Those subjects who reached criterion on the sequencing training subtest, but experienced difficulty with this subtest, fail because of the increased demand on short term memory that is specific to this subtest.

Serial Memory. In these tests, the same two stimulus elements are used, and the procedures are the same as previous subtests, except that the ISI is constant at 428 msec and the number of elements in the stimulus pattern is increased. These stimulus patterns consist of 3, 4, and 5 elements—random combinations of the two stimulus elements. The subject is initially given a stimulus pattern incorporating 3 elements, 1-1-2, for example. The experimenter demonstrates that the response panels are to be pressed three times in the order in which the stimulus elements occur. The subject is trained to wait until the entire pattern has been presented, and then make the appropriate response on the panels. Each subject begins with three-element patterns and proceeds to the next higher sequenced length once criterion has been reached. If the criterion is not reached at any sequence length, the subject is not tested further with that stimulus pair.

Same/Not Same. Those subjects who reached criterion on the sequencing training subtest, but failed to reach criterion on the sequencing with short ISIs subtest, are tested further as follows. New associations for the response panels must be learned for this subtest, so it is deferred until the end of the serial memory subtest. This test is given in order to determine whether the difficulty experienced on the sequencing with short ISIs subtest was the result of an inability to perceive the temporal sequence of the stimulus pattern, or an inability to discriminate between the stimulus items at rapid rates of presentation. The response box is turned by 90° to avoid confusion between the two subtests.

The procedure for the same/not same subtest has already been described above. It is mentioned here again because the order in which the tests are given depends on the individual subject's performance. Subjects who fail sequencing training do not go to the more complex serial memory tasks involving response panel associations to individual stimuli. So, for these subjects, the new panel associations required for the same/not same test can be taught right after the sequencing training subtest and given at that time. However, subjects who meet the criterion on sequencing training continue on to the other sequencing tasks and serial memory tasks using the same panel associations. It would cause undue confusion to teach the new associations necessary for the same/not same test right after these sequencing tests and then retrain subjects again for serial memory tests. Therefore, the same/not same test is deferred until after the serial memory subtests are completed.

It is important to note that although it is essential to give the subtests in the same order, it is not necessary to use the entire battery with each stimulus pair selected for study. The number of subtests to be given should depend on what questions one intends to answer with each stimulus pair. For example, if one merely wants to know if a subject can discriminate between two stimulus items presented in isolation, one need only give the test battery through the association subtest. If it is of interest, on the other hand, to find out whether a subject can discriminate between two stimulus items presented successively, it is possible to give the same/not same subtest alone. However, it is essential that if the tests are to be used to measure sequencing or serial memory performance, then each subtest preceding these measures must be given in the described order using the Repetition Method.

EXPERIMENTAL RESULTS

In each experiment, whether auditory or visual, verbal or nonverbal, the same general experimental method was used. The results of our initial studies are described below. The same groups of twelve carefully selected children with specific language delay and twelve normal matched controls participated as subjects in the initial studies. The criterion for inclusion as language delayed and a detailed clinical description of these subjects was given in a previous publication by Tallal and Piercy.[23] The results of the first study by Tallal and Piercy demonstrated that the language delayed children were impaired in their ability to perceive the temporal sequence of rapidly presented auditory nonverbal signals.[23] This finding confirmed the work that was reviewed above. However, we also found that these children also had equal difficulty in discriminating between the two tones in the stimulus pair when they were presented rapidly, as they had been in the sequencing condition. Thus, the sequencing deficit was the result of a more primary discrimination deficit. If one cannot discriminate between two stimuli, then one will not be able to determine their order. This deficit was demonstrated by systematically varying the duration of the inter-sound-interval (ISI) between two complex nonverbal tones of constant duration presented in sequence.

In a second experiment, Tallal and Piercy[23] tested the same language delayed and control subjects for their ability to perceive other sequences of nonverbal stimuli in the auditory and the visual modality. Performance was studied as a function of the duration of stimulus elements, the interval between elements, and the number of elements in a sequence. The results of this study showed that there were no significant differences between the two groups on any of the visual tests. On the auditory test, however, the language impaired subjects, but not the controls, were adversely affected by a decrease in the duration of the stimulus elements, by a decrease in the interval between elements, and by an increase in the number of elements. Further analysis showed that the total duration of the stimulus patterns (tone and ISI) were very highly correlated with the performance of these children. These same children could respond to two- and three-element sequences correctly at slow rates of presentation, but were unable to respond correctly to the same nonverbal stimuli when they were presented at more rapid rates. It was suggested that children with developmental language delay are incapable of responding correctly to acoustic information that is presented at rapid rates; there is a possibility that this auditory perceptual impairment may underlie their language impairment.

How could such a defect in processing rapidly changing acoustic information affect the speech perception abilities of language delayed children? Recent work in speech synthesis and perception has shown that vowels and certain consonants are processed differently by normal listeners. These differences in speech perception can be attributed to the differential duration of the critical formant information for these two classes of speech sounds, as well as to their differently shaped formants. Liberman and his colleagues[24] have shown that for the stop consonants there appears to be a relatively complex relationship between the speech sound and its acoustic representation. The essential acoustic cue for such signals is the rapidly changing spectral transitions of the second and third formants. These cues are not only transitional in character, but also are of a relatively short duration, approximately 50 msec. In contrast, the major acoustic cues for the synthetic vowels most often used in perceptual experiments are the steady-state frequencies of the first three formants; they have a relatively long duration, approximately 250 msec, and remain constant over the entire duration of the stimulus.

The results of our previous experiments demonstrated that, unlike normal children, children with developmental language delay were unable to respond correctly to nonverbal stimuli that were presented at rapid rates. On the other hand, they responded adequately to the same stimuli at slower rates of presentation. In one experiment it was demonstrated that if the duration of the tone stimuli was at least 250 msec, language delayed children could indicate which two- and three-element patterns they perceived, as well as their matched controls.

The hypothesis, that impaired auditory processing of rapidly changing acoustic cues in speech is a primary disability of language impaired children, was tested further. It was predicted that these children would be unimpaired in discriminating steady-state vowels—such as /ɛ/ (as in bed) and /æ/ (as in bad)—that were the same duration as the nonverbal steady-state tones studied previously. But, these same children would show impaired discrimination of synthesized stop consonants—such as /ba/ (as in body) and /da/ (as in dot)—that have the same *total* duration as the vowel stimuli (250 msec), but also have an initial transitional component of only 40 msec. Recall that this initial transitional component is critical for discrimination.

The same subjects and procedures used in the previous experiments were used again in this series. Two additional experiments were done: one using synthesized vowels, and another using synthesized stop consonants. Tallal and Piercy[25] reported that the ability of language impaired subjects to discriminate the vowel stimuli did not differ significantly from their discrimination of nonverbal auditory stimuli of the same duration on any of the perceptual or serial memory tasks studied. Clearly, their discrimination performance does not deteriorate as a consequence of changing from nonverbal to verbal auditory stimuli when both are of equal duration and of a steady-state character. However, the results with synthesized stop-consonants were entirely different. The language delayed subjects' discrimination of consonant stimuli was significantly inferior to both their own discrimination of vowel and nonverbal stimuli, and that of their matched controls.

Further experiments by Tallal and Piercy[26] showed that the limiting factor underlying the inferior performance of these language disordered children on the consonant tasks was the duration of the rapidly changing initial portion of the acoustic spectrum for stop consonants. In these experiments, a speech synthesizer was used to extend the initial formant transitions of the same stop consonants (/ba/ and /da/) from 40 to 80 msec; the total length of the stop consonant stimulus was maintained at 250 msec. The ability of language disordered children to discriminate between those consonants that incorporated longer transitions was found to be unimpaired. In contrast to the previous experiment in which only two of the twelve language delayed children responded adequately to the stop consonant vowel syllables with a 40 msec duration transition, all twelve children responded correctly to the same syllables with the extended duration transitions. It is important to note that normal children still perceived these extended consonants as /ba/ and /da/.

If a primary cause of the observed language disorder of some language delayed children was a failure to perceive certain speech sounds, then it would seem that these same speech sounds would be produced incorrectly or omitted in their speech. In collaboration with Dr. Rachel Stark and Barbara Curtis, this hypothesis was investigated.[27] The developmental dysphasic children who participated in speech perception studies described above, also participated as subjects in these speech production studies. These dysphasic children and twelve matched control children were tested for their ability to imitate. The imitated stimuli included: (1) isolated steady-state vowels, like /ɛ/ and /æ/;* (2) stop-consonants in consonant-vowel (CV) nonsense syllables like /bɛ/ (as in bed) and /dɛ/ (as in dead); (3) stop consonants in consonant-vowel-consonant (CVC) nonsense syllables like /bɛk/ (rhymes with deck) and /dɛg/ (rhymes with peg); and (4) stop consonants in clusters like /blɛ/ (as in blend) and /prɛ/ (as in press). These stimuli were produced by the examiner. Next, subjects were required to produce the names of objects that were pictured individually on cards. These included: (1) single syllable words with stop consonants in the initial and final positions, (such as bed or cup); (2) words primarily composed of vowels (as in eye or ear); and (3) words with dipthongs and nasals (like knife and nose). All of the subjects' responses were recorded on magnetic tape and later transcribed phonetically by two independent listeners.

The data obtained on these imitation tasks were analyzed. The overall percentage of production errors made on four classes of speech sounds was computed. These four classes—isolated vowels, nasals, stop consonants, and stop consonants in clusters—progressively incorporate more rapidly changing acoustic spectra. The results showed that the control children were able to produce all four of these classes of speech sounds equally well. The dysphasic children produced isolated vowels within normal limits in accordance with their perception of these speech sounds previously tested. However, their production of stop consonants, both singly and in clusters, was grossly impaired.

These findings suggest that the speech production of dysphasic children mirrors their speech perceptual abilities. Those speech sounds that characteristically incorporate rapid spectral changes, which are critical for their perception, are most difficult for dysphasic children to perceive, and are also most often misproduced by these children. This result adds further support to the hypothesis that some developmental language delays result, at least in part, from a primary nonverbal auditory perceptual deficit. This deficit precludes normal speech perception which, in turn, disrupts the normal development of speech and language.

*It should be remembered that these are *not* acoustically the same as vowels in word contexts; such vowels rarely reach the steady-state spectral pattern we are talking about here.

The results of Tallal and Piercy's[23, 25, 26] perceptual studies, thus far reported, were obtained with the same small groups (control and experimental subjects) of British children. It was important to determine to what extent they might be representative of other groups of language delayed children. Therefore, in collaboration with Rachel Stark, many of the same experiments were undertaken with a much larger group of very carefully selected language delayed children in America. Thirty-six language delayed children and thirty-six matched control children between the ages of five and nine participated. The results reported above were replicated with this new group of subjects.

In addition, several more studies were done to further delineate the nature of the perceptual disorder in these children. For example, in a previous study by Tallal and Piercy,[25] language delayed children were unimpaired in their ability to discriminate between 250 msec duration steady-state vowels. However, these same children were unable to respond adequately to brief duration, steady-state vowel segments of 40 msec when these segments were followed immediately by a different, longer steady-state vowel within a syllable, as in the diphthong-like stimuli used by Tallal and Piercy.[26] Furthermore, Tallal, Stark, and Curtis[27] reported that these same language delayed children's speech production abilities mirrored their speech perception abilities. Therefore, these children were impaired in producing stop consonants and consonant clusters both within nonsense syllables and real words, but were unimpaired in producing isolated steady-state vowels. It was noted in those studies that the language delayed children were impaired in producing vowels that were embedded in a syllable or word context. In such contexts, the steady-state formant values of the vowels are seldom realized. In order to investigate the perception of vowels in more detail an additional experiment was performed.

In this experiment, the ability to discriminate between two brief (40 msec) isolated steady-state vowels was investigated. In this study the results show that there were no significant differences between the language delayed and normally developing children in their ability to respond correctly to these brief signals. So it seems that language delayed children do not have difficulty responding correctly to all types of brief signals. They are unimpaired in responding correctly to isolated steady-state signals, even when they are very brief. Rather, these children seem to have particular difficulty in responding adequately to signals in which brief acoustic cues are preceded or immediately followed by other acoustic cues, as within a syllable, word, or sentence context. This was the case regardless of whether stimuli were verbal or nonverbal. Studies incorporating several other phoneme contrasts that rely on other types of temporal and spectral cues, were also investigated. The results of these other studies, in general, reflected this same pattern of perceptual disability.

We can now hypothesize that these children do not seem to have difficulty perceiving steady-state acoustic stimuli, regardless of their duration, when they are presented in isolation. However, they have marked difficulty perceiving acoustic cues that are presented either simultaneously or in close succession with others. There are a few recent findings by other authors that support this hypothesis.

Kornet, Thal, and Maxon[28] reported that dysphasic children were unimpaired in their temporal integrative functioning. In their study, the relationship between stimulus duration and stimulus intensity was examined. They found that the dysphasic subjects demonstrated threshold-duration shifts similar to those of normal subjects. The authors concluded that this indicates that dysphasic subjects are capable of responding to short duration stimuli, provided that appropriate increases in intensity are made, in the same manner as normal subjects. In this study, the brief duration pure tones used were presented singly at various intensities. At no time were two stimuli presented either simultaneously or in close succession. Therefore, according to our hypothesis, these children should not have had difficulty with this task. The results of the study indicate their response was normal.

In another recent study, using quite a different method, more evidence can be found to support our hypothesis. Tobey, Cullen, and Gallagher[29] reported that children with auditory processing disorders showed no difference in comparison to normals in ear advantage on a dichotic listening test. That is, both groups of children exhibited slight right ear advantages on a dichotic listening test using consonant-vowel syllables. However, the overall performance of the children with auditory processing disorders was significantly poorer than that of the normal children. Furthermore, the children with auditory processing disorders were able to get far fewer double correct trials than the normals. That is, when two stimuli were presented simultaneously, these children were unable to perceive both of them correctly as often as normals did. This result again suggests that there is a difficulty in processing multiple acoustic cues presented either simultaneously or in rapid succession.

One other possibility should be noted; all of the results presented in this chapter might reflect difficulties with backward or forward masking mechanisms. This question will be the emphasis of our future studies with language delayed children.

CONCLUSION

The intention of this chapter is not to suggest that all language delayed children show the same pattern of auditory perceptual deficits or that such deficits are a necessary and/or sufficient cause of the disorder. Instead, it is our purpose to demonstrate that by investigating the acoustic aspects of the speech stream in a systematic and detailed manner, consistent data can be obtained that might further our understanding of how speech and language are processed and how auditory processing contributes to this process. Furthermore, this line of research may help determine which aspects of acoustic and phonetic analysis are critical for normal language development. In conclusion, it is our hope that auditory perceptual and speech perceptual research will lead to a better understanding of some types of developmental language disabilities which, in turn, might lead to improved diagnosis and treatment for these children.

REFERENCES

1. Broadbent DE: Division of function and integration of behavior, in Schmitt FO, Worden FG (eds): The Neurosciences: Third Study Program. Cambridge, MIT Press, 1974
2. Blesser B: Discussion: Perceptual and cognitive strategies, in Stark RE (ed): Sensory Capabilities of Hearing-Impaired Children. Baltimore, University Park Press, 1975
3. Ewing AG: Aphasia in Children. London, Oxford University Press, 1930
4. Rosenthal WS, Wohlert KL: Masking level differences (MLD) effects in aphasic children. Paper presented at the American Speech and Hearing Association Convention, Detroit, Michigan, 1973
5. Milner B: Interhemispheric differences in the localization of psychological processes in man. Br Med Bull 27:272–277, 1971
6. Danaher EM, Pickett JM: Some masking effects produced by low frequency vowel formants in persons with sensorineural loss. J Speech Hear Res 18:261–271, 1975
7. Benton AL: Developmental aphasia and brain damage. Cortex 1:40–52, 1964
8. Monsees EK: Aphasia in children: Diagnosis and education. Volta Review 59:392–414, 1957
9. Hardy WG: On language disorders in young children. A reorganization of thinking. J Speech Hear Disord 8:3–16, 1965
10. Eisenson J: Developmental aphasia: A speculative view with therapeutic implications. J Speech Hear Disord 33:3–13, 1968
11. Poppen R, Stark J, Eisenson J, et al: Visual sequencing performance of aphasic children. J Speech Hear Res 12:288–300, 1969
12. Eisenson J: Aphasia in Children. London, Harper and Row, 1972
13. Lowe AD, Campbell RA: Temporal discrimination in aphasoid and normal children. J Speech Hear Res 8:313–314, 1965
14. Efron R: The effect of handedness on the perception of simultaneity and temporal order. Brain 86:261–284, 1963
15. Hirsh IJ: Auditory perception of temporal order. J Acoust Soc Am 31:759–767, 1959
16. Hirsh IJ, Sherrick CE: Perceived order in different sense modalities. J Exp Psychol 62: 423–432, 1961
17. Kornet RH, Thal DJ, Maxon A: Temporal integration in dysphasic children. Unpublished paper, 1978
18. Aten J, Davis J: Disturbances in the perception of auditory sequence in children with minimal cerebral dysfunction. J Speech Hear Res 11:236–245, 1968

19. Griffiths P: Developmental Aphasia: An Introduction. London, Invalid Children Aid Association, 1972
20. Monsees EK: Aphasia in children. J Speech Hear Disord 26:83–86, 1961
21. Rosenthal WS, Eisenson J: Auditory threshold-duration functions in aphasic subjects: Implications for the interaction of linguistic and auditory processing in aphasics. Paper presented at the American Speech and Hearing Association Convention, Chicago, Illinois, November, 1971
22. Rees NW: Auditory processing factors in language disorders: The view from Procrustes' bed. J Speech Hear Disord 38:304–315, 1973
23. Talla P, Piercy M: Developmental aphasia: Impaired rate of non-verbal processing as a function of sensory modality. Neuropsychologia 11:389–398, 1973
24. Liberman AM, Cooper FS, Shankweiler D, Studdert-Kennedy M: Perception of the speech code. Psychol Rev 74:431–461, 1967
25. Tallal P, Piercy M: Developmental aphasia: Rate of auditory processing and selective impairment of consonant perception. Neuropsychologia 12:83–94, 1974
26. Tallal P, Piercy M: Developmental aphasia, the perception of brief vowels and extended stop consonants. Neuropsychologia 13:69–74, 1975
27. Tallal P, Stark R, Curtiss B: The relation between speech perception impairment and speech production impairment in children with developmental dysphasia. Brain Lang 3:305–317, 1976
28. Kornet RH, Thal D, Maxon A: Temporal interpretation in dysphasic children. The Working Papers in Experimental Speech Pathology and Audiology, Vol. VI. 1977, pp 73–94
29. Tobey EA, Cullen JK, Gallagher AF, Rampp DL: Performance of children with auditory-processing disorders on a dichotic stop-vowel identifcation task. Paper presented at the American Speech and Hearing Association Convention, Houston, Texas, 1976

Christine Sloan

6

Auditory Processing Disorders and Language Development

Research and speculation into the nature of speech and language disorders has increased significantly in the last decade due, in part, to the influence of developments in related areas such as speech acoustics and perception, linguistics, and language acquisition. One result has been a renewed interest in auditory processing and its relation to speech and language. The notion that an auditory processing deficit underlies some kinds of speech and language disorders has been a persistent theme in both the clinical and research literature for some time (see Harris[1] and Tallal, p 81 for reviews). Recently however, advances in research technologies coupled with a more thorough understanding of the structure of speech (articulatory, acoustic, and linguistic) have made auditory processing deficits more accessible to rigid experimental investigation. The studies of Tallal and colleagues are particularly promising.

Tallal and her colleagues[2-6] have demonstrated, through a series of experiments, that some children who present with speech and language disorders have difficulties in processing auditory signals of brief duration, particularly when these occur in rapid succession as in connected speech. This finding was reported for both speech and nonspeech signals. Tallal proposed that the problems in speech and language exhibited by this group could be due to a more primary auditory processing deficit (see p 81).

PROBLEMS IN IDENTIFYING AUDITORY PROCESSING DISORDERS

The dependency of language on the auditory system seems quite obvious. This relationship between auditory function and language is acutely demonstrated in the profound difficulties in learning language experienced by children who are deaf. Yet, the possibility of subtle deficits in auditory processing has been more difficult to establish. Clinical assessment of these disorders has depended largely upon the interest, skill, and ingenuity of the clinician.

There are several reasons for the lack of evidence and lack of clinical methods for diagnosing and treating auditory processing disorders. The most obvious but frequently ignored reason was expressed by Schuell[7] in her discussion of the difficulties in the differential diagnosis of aphasia in adults; that there is no such thing as a pure test or an uncomplicated process. Performance on any task involves many kinds of past and present psychologic and neurologic events. Language itself has a complicated and interrelated structure and cannot be reduced to separate testable linguistic components, particularly in the clinical setting. When a child fails to respond accurately to a given task, there usually are many possible explanations. Finding the true explanation requires knowledge of the child and the behavior in question, and the clinical expertise to elicit the substantiating evidence from a variety of formal and informal observations.

A further reason for the difficulty in assessing auditory processing disorders has been that until recently there were only gross models of how speech was perceived and how auditory perceptual mechanisms might function. Clinical descriptions of auditory disorders referred to problems in attention, association, discrimination, sequencing and figure-ground. There were no clear and precise descriptions of what these processes might be and how they contribute to speech perception and language comprehension. Indeed, many of these notions were taken from constructs used in early learning theories and models of visual perception. In the last decade, however, considerable research in speech acoustics, speech perception, and experimental phonetics, as well as developments in linguistics, have provided much more detailed descriptions of the structure of speech and language, and the possible mechanisms or processes that might underlie their use. These new developments have given clinicians a more refined and specific conceptual map with which to identify and categorize their clinical observations.

Subtle speech and language problems often elude clinical identification because of another familiar but often forgotten characteristic of language, namely, its redundancy. Cherry[8] defines redundancy as a form of addition in which a larger number of instructions are sent than are barely necessary.

Speech is highly redundant and as such, is extraordinarily resistant to distortions and disturbances of many kinds. It may be deliberately distorted in the laboratory by filtering, noise, and other interferences, and yet remain intelligible. The concept of redundancy applies to the syntactic and semantic levels of language as well.[8]

Redundancy helps explain why rehabilitation, learning how to use new or supplemental cues when the usual ones are missing or defective, is possible. It is quite possible that subtle disorders are not identified because the assessment procedures and materials used are sufficiently redundant to enable the child to perform adequately in spite of some deficit in processing. Then too, the procedures used may not test to the limits or ceiling performance of various skills, but may only ascertain performance within the defined normal limits. It is generally acknowledged among clinicians that subtle speech and language problems that are missed in early childhood sometimes present in later years as learning and reading disabilities. It is this author's experience that less severe auditory processing disorders become problematic in later years when the reading process is initiated. (see p 189, Liberman, et al, for discussion of the relationship between speech and reading.)

It is always difficult to know when an identified behavior represents a problem or impairment, especially when it is subtle and there are few norms to refer to. The complexity of language and of language learners makes diagnosis very difficult. While it is obvious that each child must be considered individually, one way to begin to identify and understand these clinical disorders further is to continue to improve the precision and specificity of clinical theories, assessment methods, and therapy.

AUDITORY PROCESSING DISORDERS DEFINED

Tallal (p 81) presents a review of studies and clinical reports of auditory processng impairments in children with language disorders. It is not the intent here to restate these findings, but rather to summarize several characteristics of these impairments that are persistent themes in the literature and in this author's experience. These particular aspects of auditory processing disorders also seem to derive logically from our current understanding of the structure of speech and the mechanisms of perception.

Sound Identification and Discrimination

Tallal and her colleagues accomplished the most impressive series of studies with her group of aphasic children.[2-6] They first confirmed what Lowe and Campbell[9] found earlier, that aphasic children could not identify the order of two successive auditory signals. Tallal and Piercy's experiments[2, 3] demonstrated that the reason that the aphasic children failed to distinguish the order of two successive sounds was that they did not perceive that the two sounds were different. Improvement in performance occurred for both difference and order discriminations when the sounds used or the inter-sound intervals were made longer.

The extensive research in speech acoustics and speech perception done in the last decade provided Tallal and her colleagues with the framework for further studies of this phenomenon. Sounds of speech occur in succession at very rapid rates, and it has been shown that the relevant acoustic information for identifying some speech sounds is contained in very brief and changing spectral transitions.[10] Because of these characteristics of speech, Tallal hypothesized that her subjects would have difficulty discriminating speech sounds because of their difficulties in discriminating brief tones. In subsequent studies[4, 5] this difficulty was demonstrated for both consonants and vowels presented in the context of syllables. When the sounds to be identified were lengthened, however, (for example, lengthening the initial transitions of the syllables /ba/ and /da/) the aphasic children could identify the sounds as well as their matched control subjects.

Difficulty in discrimination among speech sounds has long been cited as a characteristic of some language impaired children, but few studies have conclusively demonstrted this phenomenon. McReynolds,[11] using an operant paradigm and taped natural speech, obtained results showing that as a group the aphasic children took longer to learn to discriminate among CV and CVC syllables. Some of these children totally failed to learn to discriminate among the syllables in the prescribed number of learning trials.

Undoubtedly the process of identifying speech sounds—for example, hearing /b/ as /b/ each time it occurs—has many aspects including selecting the appropriate acoustic attributes, matching the input to previous patterns experienced, matching the input to previous knowledge about the contexts or probabilities of occurrence of the input, and so on. But until the precise mechanisms for sound identification and discrimination are understood, Tallal's work provides the most descriptive account of difficulties at this level.

It seems clear that one characteristic of auditory processing disorders is the difficulty in identifying and discriminating brief sounds—speech and nonspeech—when these sounds occur in succession such as in the embedded context of speech, within a syllable or a word. A key word here is *context.* Tallal and her colleagues demonstrated that their aphasic children could identify brief steady-state signals when they were presented in isolation.[4] Difficulty arose when the same signals were presented in succession, as occurs naturally in speech. A further aspect of this difficulty was the result that if the acoustic cues important for sound identification were lengthened, aphasic subjects could perform more accurately.[5] This means that the problems in sound identification and discrimination were mainly in the transmission of the important acoustic information rather than in the formation of phonetic categories derived from that information. This somewhat supports McReynolds'[11] findings that at least some of her aphasic subjects could learn the discriminations in the prescribed number of trials but the learning took longer for them than for the controls.

The significance of this finding for the treatment of auditory processing disorders is great. It also supports the notion that the problem is in the "auditory processing" domain rather than in the domain of language.

Temporal Order

Another frequently cited characteristic of auditory processing disorders is a difficulty in judging or retaining the order or sequence of sounds or larger language units. Tallal and Piercy[2, 3] showed that on the level of individual sounds, this difficulty was secondary to a more primary difficulty in distinguishing that the two sounds were different. One must perceive that two sounds are different before one can determine their order of occurrence. Previous studies of temporal ordering or sequencing failed to consider this critical point. Therefore, the question of an ordering difficulty or a sequencing problem remains to be explored and more precisely specified by further research.

The notion of temporal order, however, is an interesting one to consider particularly in relation to the structure of speech and language. From a linguistic point of view, the structure of speech and language cannot be characterized as a simple stringing together of events, sounds, words, phrases, and so forth. Rather, there is some internal organization or interdependency of the elements within all levels of linguistic structure that gives language its context-dependent nature. Context-dependency means that elements within any unit of structure (sound sequences, words, phrases or sentences) relate to one another in predictable ways determined by the rules or grammar that govern how elements are combined in that language. So any simple notion of temporal order or sequencing as a mere concatenation of elements is incompatible with this kind of organization. Probably, the errors of language that manifest as errors in the ordering of elements have a more complicated origin than has been considered by clinicians in the past.

Bruner[12] discusses this notion of context-dependency in relation to the perceptual process. He described two features of perception: categorization and veridicality or model building. The former refers to the process of selecting the correct attributes and weighing their value; the latter relates to the idea of learning to predict and to check what goes with what or how that category fits into the whole system of interrelated categories that make up our model of the world. Bruner cites research with human subjects that demonstrates how they tend to treat even random sequences of events as though they were nonindependent of each other over time and as though they were governed by dependent probabilities.

Research in speech perception and articulation has shown that this kind of context-dependency occurs at these levels as well.[13] A more detailed discussion of this aspect of the structure of speech will be presented in a later section.

Storage of the Auditory Signal

Another characteristic of auditory processing disorders seen both in children and adults is a reduction of verbal or auditory memory span. This is a very consistent finding reported in both the research and clinical literature. In some cases these problems have been attributed to poor linguistic development. So, for example, when a child fails to retain a sentence or series of words correctly, it is presumably because he did not code the linguistic information accurately or efficiently, he did not comprehend the words, or he was unfamiliar enough with the language to make retention difficult. This is obviously an important factor. However, this author has been impressed with limitations in auditory retention span that persist in children with language disorders long after language development has reached age level expectations. In addition, one can demonstrate limited auditory retention span using familiar and simple language units the children readily understand. Tallal and Piercy[4] demonstrated that dysphasic children have difficulty retaining nonverbal auditory signals.

It seems well accepted that some kind of short-term auditory storage mechanism plays a crucial role in understanding spoken language (and in producing it as well). The acoustic signal does not remain available for processing, and since language on all levels is a context-dependent structure, there must be a mechanism (perhaps operating on several levels simultaneously) that can store required lengths of the auditory signal until enough sensory information is available for categorization.[14]

Crowder[15] cites evidence for what he calls a "Precategorical Acoustic Storage" (PSA) that has a fixed spatial or numerical capacity and a limited temporal capacity. This means that there is a limit on the units of information that can be stored at any moment of time, and a limit on the length of time these can be stored. As signals are presented to this system, earlier inputs fade as new ones follow closely behind. Presumably, information from this storage system is continuously passed on to perceptual (categorization) mechanisms as well as to some feedback system under the listener's control so that selective listening is possible. Clinically, one does get the impression of a similar limited storage capacity in children with auditory processing disorders.

Crowder's PSA is a very general model of short-term auditory storage processes. How auditory memory processes function and how they relate to perceptual and linguistic processes remains to be specified by research in these areas. However, difficulties of auditory retention or memory are impressive enough to be included as a third characteristic of auditory processing disorders.

Temporal Pattern

Ongoing speech is characterized by an overall temporal pattern or rhythm that is determined by the sequences of accented and unaccented segments. It has been suggested that these rhythmic patterns are an important organizing structure for speech production and perception, and are directly related to the structure of the language as well.[14] These rhythmic patterns, if they are perceived correctly, may facilitate memory and comprehension. It has been known for some time that speech is surprisingly resistant to many kinds of distortions and spectral manipulations intended to reduce its intelligibility except those that interfere with its temporal pattern.[8] So, temporal patterns play an important role in speech recognition.

Children with auditory processing disorders or language disorders have been noted to have difficulty in identifying and reproducing both speech and nonspeech rhythmic patterns.[16, 17] It is tempting to relate these problems in temporal patterning to a more primary problem in processing the brief segments that occur in these patterns. However, discerning temporal patterns requires perceptual storage processes as well as some perceptual (or other) mechanism for grouping sequences and constructing their overall pattern (the context-dependent function).

Peters[14] points out that all studies of auditory perception are studies of temporal factors because it is the sequential patterns of sound pressure changes that provide the necessary ingredient for perception. Furthermore, the highly patterned aspect of speech seems to derive from the structure of the language. Studies have shown, however, that temporal factors also take precedence in listening to nonspeech signals such as melodies. A study by Cutting reviewed by Peters[14] showed that acoustic signals with temporal patterns such as transitions were processed differently on a dichotic listening task regardless of whether they were speech or nonspeech types. One could say that some aspects of our perceptual mechanism are uniquely adaptive for processing speech and language.

The notion of temporal pattern is presented here because it is often singled out in the literature as an important aspect of speech perception and production. It also is intimately related to the other characteristics of auditory processing mentioned here.

Summary

The four characteristics of auditory processing disorders presented are not intended to be a definitive list, nor are any of these presented as an isolated process. Too little is known about the processes of auditory perception to provide any complete picture. Nevertheless, it is the author's intent to try to specify some aspects of auditory processing that have been demonstrated clinically, and that logically relate to our current understanding of speech and perception.

It is likely that the characteristics that have been presented here are interrelated and integrated in the perceptual process. It is this author's experience, for example, that as one aspect improves in treatment, others improve along with it. Also, one can see the interaction of these aspects in the testing process. For example, strings of words with phonetic similarity are confusing and more difficult to retain in memory than are strings of dissimilar words. Providing a temporal pattern for a series of words can facilitate memory; but if the segments are too brief for recognition, the opposite effect may occur.

Peters[14] summarizes some of these interaction effects in relation to studies of temporal order. He pointed out that performance on tasks of temporal order varies with the type and duration of the signals used, and with the rate and pattern of their presentation. In general, it appears that signal durations need to be longer for the correct perception of temporal order when the signals are more complex, when the number of signals presented is increased, and when signals are presented continuously rather than as individual discrete events.

Consideration of all of these variables influencing auditory perception seems to be very important in discovering the nature of auditory processing disorders. It is also important in the clinical situation in trying to specify as precisely as possible the conditions and tasks which result in incorrect responses. Only in this way will we begin to improve clinical methods of diagnosis and treatment.

AUDITORY PROCESSING IN THE CONTEXT OF LANGUAGE DEVELOPMENT

Human language is a complex system having a definite form or structure that ultimately is a means of representing experience. Language is a system of sound-meaning correspondences. Meaning is transposed into movements of the vocal tract to produce sounds by the speaker that, in turn, are transposed again into meaning by the listener. Mattingly[18] writes that from a linguistic point of view, the speaker-hearer has to deal with two versions of an utterance: a phonetic representation (the sound pattern) and a semantic representation (the meaning). The phonetic representation relates directly to the acoustic signal, and the semantic representation relates to acquired experience or the contents of long-term memory. Forming these representations also means knowing how they relate to one another, that is, how to reconstruct one from the other. This entails knowledge of the rules that govern their structure and organization.

The task of forming the phonetic representation from the acoustic signal could be said to be the process of speech perception. Auditory processing difficulties would very likely have a direct effect on this level of language structure.

Auditory Processing and the Perception of the Phonetic Code

The English language contains forty to forty-five distinct sounds or phonemes. They are distinct because a phoneme is the minimal element of sound that distinguishes one word from another, for example, 'cat' from 'bat'. This distinction is obviously fundamental and prerequisite for the communication of meaning. This description of the sounds of a language is, however, an oversimplification. Actually, there are hundreds of variations and nuances of pronunciation that occur both among and within speakers. These variations are due in part to the individual characteristics of each speaker's vocal tract and in part to the variations imposed by the phonetic context in which specific sounds are embedded. In learning a language, one learns to perceive all variants of a particular phoneme that occur as that phoneme. This has been described as "categorical perception." In other words, the language learner develops a kind of phonetic class or scheme that groups somewhat varying acoustic events. So the phonemes that are perceived are learned perceptual categories and, therefore, are the result of some processing beyond the physical signal.

These sounds or phonemes can be described further by a small set of subphonemic features. These are dimensions along which phonemic distinctions are made in a given language.[19] So, for example, the initial phonemes in 'pat' or 'bat' are distinguished along a voicing dimension, or more precisely, along a continuum of voice onset time—the time voicing begins relative to release of the lips in the production of these sounds.

A phoneme, then, is really a composite of distinctive features acting concurrently and sequentially in a phonetic context. The composite describes the phoneme (for example, /b/ is described in articulatory features as a bilabial, voiced, plosive consonant), and also describes differences and similarities among phonemes (for example, /p/ and /b/ are similar in manner of production but different in voicing). It is important to note that not all acoustic differences in sounds are differentiated linguistically. So the process of identifying distinctive features and hence differentiating among phonemes and words in a language is a process of selecting only the relevant acoustic differences.

Miller and Nicely[20] conducted one of the earliest studies analyzing the perceptual confusions among phonemes made by normal listeners. They found that these confusions could be characterized by a distinctive feature system. That is, errors were typically among sounds with many features in common. Furthermore, they discovered that different feature dimensions were differentially affected by the various distorting listening conditions.

Since that study, many investigations have tested the theory and the validity of distinctive features.[21] It appears that not only is there some kind of perceptual reality to phonemes but also to the distinctive features as well. If the transmission of the speech signal is distorted or impaired in some way, perceptual confusions occur among sounds sharing feature dimensions. When this confusion occurs, reception of the message is likewise impaired.

Some of the earliest research in speech perception was directed towards identifying the acoustic features within the speech signal that contributed to the recognition of individual phonemes. In other words, it was intended to find the physical reality for these linguistic distinctions. What this research discovered was that the continuous speech signal cannot be segmented into acoustic units that correspond to phonemic segments. Phonemes are not joined together acoustically; acoustic cues for successive phonemes overlap in the signal so that two or more are represented simultaneously on the same segment of sound.[13] Furthermore, the particular acoustic cue that contributed to the identification of a particular phoneme could change in different phonetic contexts; similarly, the same acoustic cue could be identified as different phonemes in different phonetic environments.[10]

So it seems that the perception of speech involves more than the simple selection of certain acoustic features from the signal. Because these features change and because they are dependent upon the context, the relevant acoustic information for phonemic segments can only be specified over time and relative to the particular context.[13]

The complexity that is involved in constructing the phonetic structure of language would seem to present very specific problems for children with auditory processing disorders. First, that child may have difficulty isolating the acoustic cues that occur in speech and are necessary for its recognition. Second, because this perceptual process is integrated with the knowledge of phonetic rules that is developing, this child would be further impaired in developing the phonologic system and in using it to guide perception. Finally, the child's difficulties in storing and patterning successive auditory signals would add a further strain to the entire process.

Prerequisites to Language Development

Language development depends on the integrity of many systems within the child and the environment. Auditory processing is only one of these. It is not the intent here to discuss all the relevant details important to language development, but only to give some overview that suggests the role of auditory processing in this general context.

H. Sinclair de-Zwart[22] has presented four prerequisites to language development: (1) the idea of communication, (2) the capacity for representation, (3) sensorimotor experience, and (4) the ability to appreciate patterns. These seem to provide a good general framework in which to view the role of auditory processing. The following is the author's elaboration.

The idea of communication. The reciprocal interactions between the infant and parent probably contribute significantly to the development of the idea of communication in the infant: the idea of relating to a world outside himself. Communication depends on the development of a sense of self and of other, and the development of language comes out of this relationship. The absence of this development and its corresponding effect on language development is acutely visible in autistic and psychotic children.

Sound is part of the relationship between infant and parent from the earliest stages. Voice qualities and vocal tones (especially the mother's) are differentiated early. Sound is part of the outside world with which the infant actively interacts in developing a sense of self and other. However, processing auditory information, although a part of this complex of communication, does not seem to be the significant factor in this first prerequisite.

The capacity for representation. The capacity for representation is the notion of developing a model of the world, learning symbols that literally "re-present" the world for the child. The child develops ways of representing experience to himself and language is one form of representation. Words stand for things, and utterances express all kinds of experiences and relationships. Obviously not all of experience is represented in language, and a child must learn what aspects of his world are coded by the language as well as how they are organized in the language structure. For example, events are most typically described in the agent-action-object form in English.

The capacity for representation seems to involve the ability to form classes or concepts (schemes according to Piaget) and to operate on those classes and determine their relationships. From this point of view, this prerequisite relates to the importance of cognitive development to language acquisition. The important point here seems to be that one must be able to organize the world in systematic ways before one can begin to label it.

Sensorimotor experience. Sensorimotor experience might be said to be the basis for all other prerequisites. One could say that it provides the raw material with which the infant develops his abilities and his resultant knowledge of the world. This experience includes direct sensory input and feedback from actions as well. In other words, the infant is not a passive recipient of information from the outside world, but is actively engaged with the world. This interaction, according to Piaget, develops into a more and more sophisticated understanding of the world.

Part of the child's sensorimotor experience is his language experience—the language he hears and the experience he receives from his own attempts to produce it. The idea here is that this experience is necessary to learning. However, if the child's auditory experience is plentiful but defective in some way, reproducing that experience alone may not be sufficient to result in accurate learning of the language code.

The ability to appreciate patterns. The final prerequisite, the ability to appreciate patterns, seems the most significant to this discussion of auditory processing disorders and language. Bruner's discussion of perception seems relevant here.[12] He writes that perception involves an act of categorization. When we are stimulated by some input, we respond by referring that input to some class of things or events. Those classes develop from our experience with certain defining attributes, repeatable and predictable patterns that come to define that category.

The child who experiences difficulty appreciating patterns cannot always identify the defining attributes, and cannot begin to develop accurate predictions or inferences about how attributes combine in various ways to form consistent patterns. The child who cannot pattern the auditory world accurately, that is, who cannot find the phonemes and their patterns of combination, will have a very difficult time learning to understand and use language. The previous discussion of auditory processing and the phonetic structure of language seems to be relevant to this prerequisite of language development.

AUDITORY PROCESSING DISORDERS: A SUBCLASS OF LANGUAGE DISORDERS

One can look at language development as a composite of many functions and aspects of the child's experience. Language disorders, too, can be related to many aspects of the child and the environment. The renewed interest in language disorders in the past few years has resulted in a proliferation of theories, research techniques, testing materials, and evaluation procedures. All of these measures have been successful in defining and identifying this population, and in bringing their special needs to the attention of speech clinicians, special educators, and physicians. The identity of this population seems well established. However, the nature and cause of these disorders are still uncertain. No test has been developed that can differentiate among this population. Most likely several causes and types of problems exist.

Clinicians are usually impressed by the variety of patterns apparent in observing language behavior, in testing, and in the history information obtained from an evaluation. The clinician's role is to somehow identify common threads or repeatable patterns that suggest the main cause or underlying deficit producing the observed behavior. Following this, the clinician plans a treatment program. Ideally there is some relationship between the underlying problem and the treatment administered so that therapy is not aimed at isolated symptoms or behaviors, but has an overall effect on language development.

This approach can be difficult to realize. It is sometimes easier to treat all language problems alike with the usual language programs available for therapy. These approaches are obviously appropriate for many children, and they may be beneficial to most children with language disorders. But one must be careful to avoid allowing subtle problems in processing that involve finer levels of discrimination to remain. It is important to assess all levels of language structure carefully beginning with the most simple sound discriminations.

Not all language disorders are characterized by an auditory processing disorder as it has been described here. One example is the child who imitates or echos speech very well but without comprehending meaning. This child seems to be structuring the auditory signal into phonetic patterns as evidenced by his ability to reproduce them. His problems relate to other levels of language structure, and to the integration of these with the sound pattern.

On the other hand, an auditory processing disorder can affect the overall development of language. Not only is the development of phonetic structure and speech affected, but the development of grammar and semantic relations can be deficient as well. Meaning and syntactic constituent information is associated with sound patterns as well, particularly with stress, intonation, and juncture. So the development of meaning and its expressions in the sentences of the language are fundamentally linked to the ability to process auditory signals. In addition, limitations in auditory retention span would seem to have an effect on the understanding and production of sentences, particularly complex structures such as those containing a number of embedded elements.

In summary, auditory processing disorders are a type of language disorder in children. In evaluating and treating language disorders it is important to determine the exact nature of the problems contributing to the language behavior so that the treatment plans developed will be most effective. Furthermore, it is important that clinicians continue to refine their testing and treatment skills so that they can contribute to the understanding of these types of impairments.

AUDITORY PROCESSING DISORDERS AND READING

Liberman, Shankweiler, and colleagues (p 189) hypothesize that the process of reading is closely related to the speech system, that is, to the knowledge the child has about the phonologic structure of his language. There is much to support this notion. This author's experience in evaluating and treating reading disabilities in children would support this further. Many of these children have difficulty discriminating among speech sounds, and they seem to be completely unaware that the letters of the printed word have some relationship to the spoken sounds of the words. In fact, a major goal of treatment is the ability to segment the sound stream into its phonetic elements. For many children this understanding seems to develop or be present with very little direct instruction. But for others, this connection is not made, and may be difficult to acquire. Liberman, *et al.* have shown that this ability is associated with early reading achievement.

Reading disabilities are mentioned here because it is this author's experience that children with auditory processing disorders are potential candidates for reading disabilities when they become school age, and, that the appropriate intervention before this time may help to reduce that possibility. It is also this author's impression that mild forms of auditory processing disorders may not be detectable in early childhood, especially in the child with other good language skills, but may manifest themselves later in reading difficulties.

SUMMARY

This discussion was intended to bring together what is known about auditory processing disorders in children with what is known about the aspects of language that are most directly affected by these kinds of problems. This is intended to be open-ended and not conclusive. We can continue to refine and specify further the nature of these disorders by bringing together our clinical observations with the outcomes of our theories and research.

REFERENCES

1. Harris C: Language disorders: Some answered questions. Communicative Disorders: An Audio Journal for Continuing Education 2, New York, Grune and Stratton, March, 1977
2. Tallal P, Piercy M: Defects of non-verbal auditory perception in children with developmental aphasia. Nature 241:468–469, 1973
3. Tallal P, Piercy M: Development aphasia: Impaired rate of nonverbal processing as a function of sensory modality. Neuropsychologia 11:389–398, 1973
4. Tallal P, Piercy M: Developmental aphasia: Rate of auditory processing and selective impairment of consonant perception. Neuropsychologia 12:83–93, 1974
5. Tallal P, Piercy M: Developmental aphasia: The perception of brief vowels and extended stop consonants. Neuropsychologia 13:69–74, 1975
6. Tallal P: Perceptual and linguistic factors in the language impairment of developmental aphasics: An experimental investigation with the Token Test. Cortex 11:196–205, 1975
7. Schuell H, Jenkins JJ: The nature of language deficit in aphasia. Psychol Rev 66:45–67, 1959
8. Cherry C: On Human Communication. Cambridge, M.I.T. Press, 1957, pp 186–187
9. Lowe AD, Campbell RA: Temporal discrimination in aphasoid and normal children. J Speech Hear Res 8:313–314, 1965
10. Liberman AM, Cooper FS, Shankweiler DP, et al: Perception of the speech code. Psychol Rev 74:431–461, 1967
11. McReynolds LV: Operant conditioning for investigating speech sound discrimination in aphasic children. J Speech Hear Res 9:519–528, 1966
12. Bruner JS: On perceptual readiness. Psychol Rev 64:123–152, 1957
13. Shankweiler D, Strange W, Verbrugge R: Speech and the problem of perceptual constance, in Shaw R, Bransford J (eds): Perceiving Acting and Knowing. Hillsdale, N.J., Lawrence Erlbaum Associates, 1977, pp 315–346
14. Peters R: The measurement of temporal factors in auditory perception, in Singh S (ed): Measurement Procedures in Speech, Hearing, and Language. Baltimore, University Park Press, 1975, pp 157–175
15. Crowder RG: Visual and auditory memory, in Kavanagh JR, Mattingly IG (eds): Language by Ear and by Eye. Cambridge, M.I.T. Press, 1972, pp 251–275
16. Aten J, Davis J: Disturbances in the perception of auditory sequence in children with minimal cerebral dysfunction. J Speech Hear Res 11:236–245, 1968
17. Griffiths P: Developmental Aphasia: An Introduction. London, Invalid Children Aid Association, 1972
18. Mattingly IG: The human aspect of speech, in Kavanagh JF, Cutting JE (eds): The Role of Speech in Language. Cambridge, M.I.T. Press, 1975, pp 63–72
19. Jakobson R, Fant CG, Halle M: Preliminaries to Speech Analysis. Cambridge, M.I.T. Press, 1952
20. Miller GA, Nicely PE: An analysis of the perceptual confusions among some English consonants. J Acoust Soc Am 27:338–352, 1955
21. Singh S: Distinctive Features: Theory and Validation. Baltimore, University Park Press, 1976, pp 101–152
22. Sinclair-de Zwart H: On pre-speech. Paper presented at the Sixth Child Language Research Forum, Stanford University, Palo Alto, 1974

Christine Sloan

7

Auditory Processing Disorders in Children: Diagnosis and Treatment

Auditory processing disorders are part of the general category of language disorders in children. The specific deficits characterizing this clinical group affect all levels of linguistic development but have the most significant impact on the development of the phonetic structure of the langugage. (see p 101 for a more detailed discussion.) The problems associated with auditory processing disorder include

1. Difficulty perceiving the accurate acoustic cues for the identification of speech sounds, especially when these are embedded in the contexts of syllables, words or phrases
2. Difficulty retaining a sequence of auditory signals
3. Difficulty organizing phonemes into accurate sequential patterns both in perception and in production
4. Difficulty perceiving the temporal patterns of speech and utilizing these to facilitate recognition and retention

The child with an auditory processing disorder will "misperceive" sounds, words, and phrases. It is possible that some brief sound segments are not detected at all. Longer auditory messages are not retained in their entirety, or they may be missed altogether. This limitation in retention span also interferes with the accurate reception and comprehension of language. These children are severly affected when speech is presented at rapid rates. They cannot reconstruct the phonetic structure of an utterance from such a rapid influx of acoustic information. Perhaps because of this the development of the phonologic system is directly affected.

Auditory processing disorders are problems in the accurate and efficient transmission of acoustic information important to speech perception; they have a secondary effect on the development of articulation and language as well. Because it is primarily a perceptual problem, the evaluation of auditory processing disorders is directed toward assessing how the child processes auditory messages at all levels—sounds, syllables, words, and connected utterances. It is also important to evaluate how well the child has developed the phonetic structure of his language as it is reflected in his perception and production of phonetic segments and sequences. Treatment is aimed toward improving perceptual processes so that they become accurate and efficient. The assumption underlying this treatment approach is that as perceptual processing improves and accurate acoustic information is transmitted to language processes, normal language development will occur.

IDENTIFYING THE PROBLEM

There is no test for auditory processing disorders. There are many tests that present stimuli primarily through the auditory modality (receptive language tests, auditory language comprehension tests, speech sound discrimination tests, auditory retention tests), but none is comprehensive enough to provide a basis for differential diagnosis. Furthermore, too many factors enter into any testing situation and contribute to the child's success or failure so that the likelihood that a single test will distinguish auditory processing disorders is very small.

The best means of evaluation and diagnosis is to assess the child with a variety of speech and language instruments that focus on different aspects of speech, language, and auditory function. In addition, it is important to make careful observations of the child's spontaneous behavior and a report of its history. It is more important to look at the qualitative aspects of the child's responses, than at any score *per se*. A score may have value as a reference for comparison later, but the immediate goal of evaluation is to understand how the child is processing the situation before him.

Typical Patterns of Performance on Speech and Language Tests

There is no single overall profile of performance that can characterize the child with an auditory processing disorder. An auditory processing disorder can exist in a child who has no other apparent problems, even with language, other than those produced by the primary deficit. On the other hand, the auditory disorder can be part of a complex of problems relating to speech and language development. Although some tasks (sound discrimination and auditory retention, for example) will always be performed with difficulty in this population, other language tasks may be performed well. This is because those other aspects of language development that are not imparied continue to develop, resulting in improved scores on language tests as the child grows. Recall that language is highly redundant; the child learns to use the cues available to him, compensating for those that are absent or less accessible.

This is particularly true when the auditory processing disorder is not severe, or when it manifests in a child who is very adept with language. These children may not be identified until the introduction of reading places increased demands on their abilities to process and extract phonetic elements. (See p 189 for a detailed discussion of the relationship between reading and the phonetic structure of the language.)

Despite the fact that the overall pattern or profile of performance on speech and language tests may be variable among children with auditory processing disorders, there are some characteristics of their test behavior that recur and provide evidence for diagnosis. These characteristics and patterns will be discussed below.

SCATTER

As in the case of other specific learning disabilities, children with auditory processing disorders usually present with a wide scatter of scores on speech and language test batteries (like the *Illinois Test of Psycholinguistic Abilities*[1] or the *Detroit Tests of Learning Aptitude*,[2] for example). Some scores may be near age level while others may fall far below. In this author's experience, certain measures are more likely to be near age level than others; for example, vocabulary tests like the *Peabody Picture Vocabulary Test*.[3] This test is simple to perform. Response choices are provided from which the child can choose. The child can control the rate at which words are presented somewhat, by the speed with which he responds, and there is no penalty for repetition. This type of measure usually is the first to show improvement when therapy is initiated.

Performance on measures of language comprehension will be more variable with some children doing poorly and others doing well. A test like the *Test for Auditory Comprehension of Language*[4] may show a mixed picture: the vocabulary items may be correct even to the highest age level, while the items presented with sentence length stimuli (especially those contrasting brief elements like 'is' and 'are') may be in error, even the developmentally easier ones. It is very helpful to examine a test protocol to see if a pattern emerges in the types of items that were passed and failed.

Language tests that have an open-ended format, like the General Information subtest of the *Peabody Individual Achievement Tests*,[5] are most difficult, especially if they require specific responses (and the corresponding specific phonetic patterns for these) and provide no additional cues or choices. This particular subtest also asks for information using lengthy descriptions which creates additional demands for accurate auditory retention. It is helpful to administer several language tests having different formats and to compare the results obtained. The differences in performance can be considered in light of the processing demands inherent in each of the tests.

Performance on tests of auditory memory is typically low whether digits, words, or sentences are used. Usually the performance remains the same whether the series is presented slowly with equal stress on each element, or in a rhythm of stressed and unstressed elements. In the first case, the demand seems to be greater on auditory storage processes; in the later case, there is the need to perceive and reproduce the temporal pattern.

Several other patterns can be identified in imitation, articulation, sound discrimination and grammar that will be discussed further.

IMITATION

Tests employing imitation responses are particularly revealing (like the *Carrow Elicited Language Inventory,*[6] for example). One can analyze the responses on this test not only in terms of linguistic elements (for which it was intended), but also with regard to the acoustic dimensions inherent in the sentence stimuli. For example, errors can be evaluated in terms of the acoustic duration; children with auditory processing disorders will omit, shorten, or substitute the short unstressed elements within the sentences. These could be sounds, syllables, or whole words. This author treated one child who typically omitted short unstressed segments or substituted the neutral vowel /ə/ for syllables and short words.

Of course, on language imitation tasks as well as in spontaneous language production, perceptual and linguistic factors will interact. It is important to have a thorough understanding of the sequence of normal language development in order to determine whether the response pattern observed can be explained by predictions from normal language development, or must be considered to reflect some specific error in processing.

Imitation responses provide one of the few indirect glimpses of the child's perceptual experience. If the child understands how to imitate and if his articulatory mechanism operates normally, we can tentatively assume that the speech he produces reflects, at least in part, the speech he perceives.

ARTICULATION

Tallal, Stark, and Curtiss[7] examined the articulation of their children with auditory processing disorders and found that production of sounds mirrored perception. A very careful assessment of articulation is important to the evaluation of auditory processing disorders.

Articulation should be tested in the usual way (picture tests that include all the individual phonemes in all positions in words), and also in spontaneous speech. One should be aware of the following patterns: (1) inaccurate production of short vowels; (2) omissions of the stop consonants; (3) failure to distinguish phonemes by voicing, especially the stops; (4) a pattern of errors that is not consistent with the developmental acquisition of articulation (developmentally early sounds may not be stable while later ones are); and (5) very unintelligible speech that one finds extremely difficult to analyze along any phonetic dimensions. The prosody of speech may also seem somewhat unusual. Speech may have a somewhat staccato quality; there may be few words produced with more than one main stressed syllable.

Articulation mirrors perception. The pattern of articulation errors should be analyzed in terms of the acoustic characteristics of each sound and of sequences of sounds that form the words and phrases transcribed. Older children with relatively intelligible speech may seem to have little difficulty in articulation. However, if one listens very closely, one sometimes hears considerable variability in the production of certain phonetic features, especially voicing. A sample of their productions of /p/ and /b/, for example, might reveal that they do not have very stable phonemic categories that clearly distinguish these two sounds along that dimension. One hears sounds that are somewhere in between the two, that is, that sound a little bit like both of them.

SOUND DISCRIMINATION

There are several tests designed to assess how well the child can differentiate between words and sounds that are acoustically similar, or how well the child can listen and discriminate under various distracting conditions (the *Wepman Test of Auditory Discrimination*[8] and the *Goldman-Fristoe-Woodcock Test of Auditory Discrimination*,[9] for example). These kinds of tests can be helpful in identifying and validating an auditory processing problem, but a more specific and simplified exploration of sound discrimination ability based on distinctive feature contrasts is usually more helpful to understanding the problem and providing data that can be used in planning treatment.

One method for evaluting how well the child is perceiving the important acoustic differences among individual speech sounds is to set up a discrimination learning situation using related pairs of sounds that are distinguished along a single feature dimension (like /p/ and /b/, or /m/ and /n/). The sounds can be associated with their letters and with different colors to reinforce their difference. The clinician then associates the sound and its letter repeatedly, perhaps lengthening its production and repeating frequently until the child can make the distinction (visual and tactile cues can also be added). Then the sounds are presented singly in random order and at a normal speaking rate to see if the child can identify them accurately. Correct responses are reinforced. The clinician can observe whether the child can make the discrimination, and how quickly he learns to do so. If the clinician suspects that the child does not distinguish some whole words, these can be evaluated using the same format.

It is important to ascertain not only if the child can identify the sounds, but also if he can do so with certainty, quickly, and without hestiation. We are interested in the accessibility of processing functions as well as their accuracy.

A very young child (under five years old) may not be able to understand and respond to this format. For this child, or for older children who are confused by the two-choice method, another approach can be tried. This is similar to the technique used by Kuhl (p 35) to evaluate sound discrimination ability in infants. The clinician produces one of the two sounds in the related pair (/p/ and /b/, for example) repeatedly at a slow rate. Then the second sound of the pair is produced while maintaining the same tone of voice and rate of presentation. That sound is continued and then changed again to the original sound. The child is taught to signal the clinician when he hears a change. The change can be emphasized with visual cues, long durations, and other distinctions during learning trials, but the testing should be conducted using a normal speaking rate and the auditory modality alone.

EXPRESSIVE LANGUAGE

The expressive language of children with auditory processing disorders may be very similar to their imitative responses with regard to sentence structure. In each case, the patterns of the language reflect in large part the perceptual information the child is receiving. As mentioned earlier in relation to imitative responses, there can be a pattern of omissions of short unstressed segments of the sentence or word; frequently these short elements are the grammatical connectors, relational terms, auxillaries, and so on. This sometimes gives expressive language a telegraphic quality. There may also be an undifferentiated marker (the neutral vowel / ə /, for example) in place of a word or inflection.

Sometimes it is difficult to distinguish between errors of language and errors that may be the result of inaccurate processing. One child used the word 'he' for both female and male second-person pronouns. Discrimination testing demonstrated that the child did not distinguish between 'he' and 'she' in perception.

Unfortunately there are no studies that have thoroughly examined the expressive language of children with auditory processing disorders to provide a comprehensive account of the patterns they present. The clinician is left with the guidelines provided by normal language development. One can look at the language structure with those guidelines in mind and with an understanding of how perceptual processing difficulties could interfere with that process.

SUMMARY

Although there is no single overall profile of performance that distinguishes the child with auditory processing disorders, there are some characteristic patterns and deficits that identify this group. A clinician must look for the patterns that emerge in the testing data and consider both the qualitative and quantitative aspects of the child's responses. It is also helpful to evaluate the child's performance in light of what one would expect from normal speech and language development and from the presence of an auditory processing disorder.

Task Analysis

A methodology that is useful in identifying auditory processing disorders has been alluded to in the previous section and it deserves some special discussion. This is the approach of task analysis: breaking up a task into its subcomponents and the skills required to complete each component. This is a very useful approach in diagnosis. Different tasks place different demands upon the child and the various skills he has acquired, whether perceptual or linguistic. In task analysis the clinician tries to determine what the child must know and what skills he must have in order to complete the task. This is done by analyzing the task very carefully: the type and structure of the stimuli presented; the type of interaction the child has with those stimuli; and the nature of the response that is required.

Task analysis helps the clinician understand the baffling pattern of scatter usually found in the child's performance. Close analysis of the individual tests and test items may reveal that errors tended to occur when stimuli were long units of language (requiring auditory storage), or when signals were presented rapidly, or when the words were short and unstressed.

Of course, several patterns may emerge and intereact. The approach of task analysis, however, helps the clinician understand why the child performed the way he did and what characteristics of the stimuli, the responses or the test procedures contributed to success and failure. This kind of data is valuable to diagnosis and to treatment plans.

THERAPY FOR AUDITORY PROCESSING DISORDERS

The principles of therapy that are described below are based on several levels of knowledge: (1) what we know about speech and its structure; (2) what we know about perception; (3) what we know about auditory processing disorders; and (4) what this author has learned from experience. These are presented as guidelines to clinicians and not as any final program that can have general applicability. Too much is still uncertain about the nature of auditory processing disorders and their affect on language processes to offer more at this time. Each child must still be evaluated and planned for individually.

This approach to therapy is based on the definition of auditory processing disorders presented by this author: that auditory processing disorders are perceptual in nature, and that the language problems that exist are directly related to these more primary perceptual difficulties. Therapy, then, is directed toward making perceptual processes function more accurately and efficiently. Improved perceptual processing, in turn, should affect more normal development of speech and language.

It is this author's experience that auditory processing disorders can occur as isolated disabilities in children. However, they can also be part of a more pervasive speech and language disorder. In those cases, treatment must be broader than it is described here. The clinician should keep in mind the importance of working directly with the perceptual deficit; this kind of treatment will have a general effect on the whole speech and language system.

The following are several principles of treatment for auditory processing disorders. Some are well-established principles of therapy applicable to many kinds of problems. They are presented here because of their importance in this particular case. Following this list of treatment principles is a report of the use of these methods for a child with an auditory processing disorder.

Treatment Principles for Auditory Processing Disorders

Give the child direct instructions. Children should not be left to guess the objective of therapy or the goal they are seeking. Give the child very direct instructions about what he is supposed to be listening for, what he is supposed to hear, and what he is supposed to do. These directions may have to be repeated and discussed before each therapy session, and sometimes before each training trial. It may be helpful to represent the task in another modality as a further step in helping the child understand the task before him.

Don't allow Guessing. In order to facilitate signal detection, the child should be discouraged from guessing throughout the treatment program. You want to develop accuracy and certainty in the perceptual process. When children begin this kind of perceptual training process, they will want to guess. They want to have the "right" answer. It is very important to help them understand that the goal of therapy is to develop certainty—accurate identification of the signal. Progress is more rapid when the child stops guessing and works for this goal. The child should be allowed to hear the signal again, to have additional cues, or to listen to the signal under any condition that will facilitate certainty in his response. As therapy progresses, these techniques to help identification are gradually decreased but the goal of certainty should continue throughout treatment.

Maximize signal detection. This means doing whatever you can to make the signal you are working with—sound, syllable, word or phrase—perceptible for the child. Some ways to do this are (1) to prolong the signal; (2) to simplify the signal; (3) to present the signal many times (keeping rate slow to allow space for processing); and (4) to associate the critical acoustic feature with cues from other sensory modalities (for example, feedback from articulation, visual posture of the articulators, the feeling of aspiration on the hand, and so on). This may be a trial and error approach in the beginning. The important point is to find a way of presenting the signals used in training so that they can be distinguished by the child with 75 percent success.

Gradually withdraw cues. Once accurate identification or discrimination is obtained and stabilized under the maximal conditions for signal detection, the techniques one has employed to obtain this accuracy should be withdrawn one at a time. This may be an off and on process in the beginning; that is, one cue is removed in a session and in the next session it must be used again and removed again. The change may be very gradual and take some time to accomplish, particularly across sessions. In addition, each new acoustic contrast that is introduced may have to be established in this gradual way—first with maximal cues and techniques for identification and then the gradual elimination of each one in turn.

Present signals in phonetic contrasts. The child with an auditory processing disorder has not developed very stable and accurate phonetic categories. The perception of these categories seems easiest to establish through contrast, especially contrasts along a specific feature dimension. With this approach the child is learning the contrasts that distinguish the sounds of his language. An evaluation of the child's ability to identify and discriminate among sounds should provide the data for selecting phonetic contrasts to be trained, for example, vowel color (/ɛ/ vs /æ/), voicing (/t/ vs /d/), place of articulation (/b/ vs /d/), and so on. Various manipulations of these contrast pairs can be employed (as discussed previously) to maximize detection of the contrast. The contrast can be emphasized further by associating each member of the pair with a different color or letter.

Work until responses are automatic. It is not only important to teach an auditory distinction, but it is also important to make that distinction readily accessible and retrievable. This is an important aspect of therapy that is directed towards improved processing. The child's discrimination responses should become very stable and automatic. He should demonstrate success over many trials and over some length of time. Responses should be quick and certain as well as accurate. When one learned distinction is being established in this way, another contrast can be introduced at the same time so that the learning strategies developed in the first instance continue to be used.

Make the child responsible for signal detection from the start. It is very helpful to the child's progress to make him responsible for controlling the way in which signals are manipulated for detection. Encourage the child from the beginning to tell you when he needs more help, more information, or more cues to detect the signal and discriminate the contrast. For example, the child can ask for more repetitions, for a slower presentation, for prolongation of the sound, or for any cue that helps him be sure of his response. What can happen through this procedure is that the child begins to employ these strategies himself with his own speech as a means for identification. When this happens, he begins to carry a built-in method for sound identification with him all the time.

Work on several levels of phonetic structure. Auditory perceptual training can be conducted on several levels of phonetic structure at the same time. This is particularly necessary in the beginning when the child may be able to attend to very difficult listening tasks for only brief periods. A number of tasks can be used, each working with a different phonetic unit; for example, sound contrasts, identification of the number of syllables in words, or identification of specific words in phrases. This approach also provides the child with these larger contexts from the very beginning, helping him to experience the relationship between the very difficult and specific distinctive feature contrast training, and the more general situation of listening to whole utterances.

Use articulation as soon as possible. As soon as the child can imitate the sounds you are presenting for identification and discrimination, use his feedback from articulation to reinforce perception. The procedure of listen then respond is changed to listen, *repeat,* and then respond. When production and perception begin to work together, progress seems to be significantly enhanced.

Program in very small steps: From simple to more complex. In training children with auditory processing disorders to perceive minimal phonetic contrasts, we are building in the phonetic structure of the language. Their particular disability has not allowed them to do this properly. Therefore, we must use very small steps, training each consonant-vowel pair in turn, if need be. For example, we might train the contrast, /te/ and /de/, and think the child has learned to distinguish between /t/ and /d/. It may be necessary to train with these two consonants in several (or all) vowel contexts, and to do so until each becomes a readily accessible, automatic perceptual response. We are getting down to the most minimal phonetic elements we can control in the clinical setting, and systematically training the child to perceive each of these. If generalization does occur, that is fine, but do not assume that it will.

The sounds selected for training should be simple in the beginning and gradually increase in phonetic complexity. For example, one could begin with the contrast of /t/ and /d/ in one consonant-vowel context, then gradually add new vowels to the syllables for contrast, then move to a CVC word, then move to the various positions in the word, then include consonant blends, multisyllabic words, and so on. At each level you are increasing the complexity either by adding a new element or changing an existing one. Your understanding of phonetic structure can be your guide.

Use blocks of trials. In doing discrimination training it is helpful to present signals in blocks of trials; for example, ten in succession, with some rest or gap in between trials. This is helpful for record keeping and it gives the child a prescribed period of attention to tune into. This author has found it useful to work in blocks of ten trials and to represent these trials to the child in some concrete (pegs in a board) or graphic way.

Maintain a high success rate. Try to maintain an average of about 75 to 80 percent accuracy in the child's responses. When new signals are introduced, this may be difficult to obtain at once. However, if this success rate is not operative after two or three sessions, the clinician should carefully review the procedures and improve signal detection until that level of success is obtained. This is very important because this kind of training can be very tedious for the child, especially in the beginning.

Use a nondistracting but concrete reinforcement for correct responses. The reinforcement used for correct responses should not interfere with the listening set that the child develops in the course of the treatment. That is, it should be something simple (for example, putting pegs in a board) that takes a minimum of time. In this way, the block of ten trials can go along smoothly and at an even rate, and the child can maintain his listening set throughout. Also, this will allow the clinician to present as many as eight to ten trials (80 to 100 responses) in a 30-minute session.

Begin with a warm-up. The first few minutes of therapy can begin with a review, using stimuli that the child has learned to distinguish in earlier sessions. This helps the child get into the right listening set with a task at which he is successful. It also helps the child see what he has already accomplished so that he is more confident that he can master the next contrast. Sometimes in the beginning it is helpful to end the session with successful tasks as well.

Develop a simple system to keep track of quantitative and qualitative data. It is very important to keep very exact records of where a child is and the conditions used in training a phonetic contrast. It is useful to develop a code that allows you to note the conditions as well as the child's responses; for example, *R* means repetition given (or requested), *P* means prolongation given, *V* means visual cue, and so forth. The child's responses should be noted as correct or incorrect, and as prompt or delayed. This enables the clinician to see progress throughout, such as a change in condition (removing a cue) that maintains a high success rate, or a change in responses from delayed to prompt.

SUMMARY

These are some of the techniques and procedures that have been useful to this author in planning and implementing treatment programs for children with auditory processing disorders. There are many other important general therapeutic considerations that could be added. The following case description illustrates how some of these principles were put into action for one particular child.

Auditory Processing Disorder: Sixteen Months of Treatment

The following case of an auditory processing disorder was described in a previous publication.[10] Most of this report is presented here.

CASE HISTORY

This is a report of 16 months of treatment of a five-year-old girl suspected of having difficulties processing auditory signals of brief duration as described by Tallal and colleagues in their experiments.*[11-15]

*Tallal discovered that her groups of aphasic children could not process auditory signals (both speech and nonspeech) when these were presented at rapid rates. The performance of these children could be improved, however, when longer signal durations and/or longer inter-signal-intervals were used.

On initial examination the child spoke in single words, and in sentences of two to five words. Most utterances beyond one or two words in length were unintelligible to everyone but her mother. Those utterances that were intelligible were telegraphic in style in that they contained the words that carried semantic information and omitted many short unstressed grammatical or connecting words. There was a tendency for a neutral /ə/ or other short vowel sound to be produced in place of short or unstressed words and syllables.

Speech was characterized by single vowel or consonant-vowel units. Consonants were nasals or plosives differentiated by place of articulation but not by voicing. Long vowels were usually produced accurately; short vowels were more variable.

Scores on standardized tests of receptive vocabulary, language comprehension, and auditory memory were below age level. In addition, there was evidence of "misperception"—confusing words that sounded alike on verbal retention and imitation tasks. The child herself expressed her confusion in following directions and remembering instructions. There was no significant medical or developmental history. The girl's father reportedly had difficulty learning to read.

Initially this child was enrolled in a language stimulation group to develop vocabulary and language comprehension. This lasted three months and resulted in near age-level scores on pictorial tests of vocabulary and language comprehension. The overall pattern of expressive speech and difficulties in retention and directions remained the same.

It was hypothesized that this child's speech and language behavior resulted from difficulties in distinguishing auditory patterns of short duration as evidenced by: (1) the omission or reduction of short or unstressed segments in spontaneous speech and imitation; (2) the greater accuracy in production of long vowels as opposed to short vowels; (3) the omission or reduction of consonant segments in speech; (4) failure to make the voicing feature distinction; and (5) the presence of difficulties in auditory perception and retention of language.

Treatment. A treatment program was developed that involved training in making auditory discriminations that require processing cues of short duration. The clinician's live voice was used throughout. However, the presentation of auditory signals was controlled and programmed along several dimensions including: (1) signal duration; (2) presentation rate; (3) number of repetitions; and (4) phonetic complexity. In other words, training progressed from prolonged, somewhat exaggerated signal durations to durations of normal speech; from slow to more rapid presentation rates; from many signal repetitions to only one; and from simple to more complex phonetic patterns and response demands.

It should be noted that finding the right progression was an evolutionary process, somewhat intuitive and somewhat trial and error. Theories of phonetic structure, of speech perception, and of auditory processing provided a general conceptual framework. Training was conducted on the levels of individual phonemes, syllables, and words.

An outline of the phoneme discrimination program is presented in Table 7-1. The final objective of this program was the ability to perceive the individual phonetic segments of speech. The pair of cognates /t/ and /d/ were chosen to begin training.

Table 7-1
Phoneme Discrimination Program

Step 1.	Tactile cueing for /t,d/
Step 2.	Sound prolongation, /t,d/
Step 3.	Vowel variations with /t,d/
Step 4.	Word-initial positions with /t,d/
Step 5.	All word positions for /t,d/
Step 6.	Sound and place identification, /t,d/
Step 7.	Transfer to other stops, /p,b/ and /k,g/
Step 8.	Increased phonetic length and complexity
Step 9.	CVC word analysis and synthesis

Each sound was paired with the letter and with a specific color. The child responded to the presentation of one or the other sounds by pointing to the corresponding letter. Correct responses were reinforced by giving the child a peg to place in a board. A response criterion of an average of 80 percent success across trials was maintained throughout.

In *Step 1* the discrimination was established using the tactile cue of aspiration felt on the hand. Then this cue was gradually reduced *(Step 2)* and the prolonged auditory signal was presented alone. The effect of prolongation on /t/ and /d/ was an extension of the prevoicing aspiration for /t/, so that it sounded like /t^{h} ə /, and an extension of the voiced segment for /d/, so that it sounded like /^{n}d ə /. In the beginning these prolonged signals were presented at a very slow rate with repeated instructions to listen closely. The child could hear the signal as many times as she wished before responding; she was not allowed to guess. Gradually the signal duration, presentation rate, and number of repetitions were varied until the discrimination of /tə/ and /də/ was obtained at normal durations and presentation rates.

Step 3 involved changing the vowel. Interestingly, the change in vowel required altering the signal presentation again; that is, going back to the prolonged duration, slowing the presentation rate, and frequent repetitions to maintain the 80 percent success criterion. With each new vowel, however, fewer and fewer learning trials with the added cues were required.

Step 4 involved identifying /t/ and /d/ in initial word positions. *Step 5* extended the task to all word positions. *Step 6* involved making two decisions: (1) identifying the sound (/t/ or /d/); and (2) identifying its position in the word. This made the detection process more complex by requiring a search for the sound within the phonetic sequence. The task in Step 6 was made more difficult in *Step 7* by increasing the length and phonetic complexity of the words used; for example, by presenting /t/ and /d/ in consonant blends and multisyllabic words.

Step 8 involved introducing the bilabial and velar cognates /p/ and /b/, and /k/ and /g/. This might have been done sooner in the program as well. Interestingly, the discrimination of these pairs was almost immediate, unlike the laborious training with each vowel for /t/ and /d/. Other consonant pairs were introduced and distinguished very quickly.

The final step *(Step 9)* of sound training was intended to establish the ability to phonetically segment and blend CVC words with a variety of consonants and vowels. This step helped establish the preliminary skills needed to sound out words in reading.

Initially there was no direct work on *articulation*. However, the clinician periodically probed for production of /t/ and /d/. By Step 4 the child was able to imitate these sounds accurately in initial word positions about 80 percent of the time. Thereafter the child was instructed to listen, repeat, and then respond so that self-monitoring through her own articulation was encouraged.

In addition to the training in phoneme discrimination, programs were developed using the same methods to train the ability to identify the unstressed syllables in words and the unstressed words in phrases.

Results. Therapy was terminated when the phoneme discrimination program was completed. At that time, the child's speech was completely intelligible. All sounds with the exception of /r/ were produced accurately in spontaneous speech. Sentences ranged in length from 2 to 16 words with a mean of 6.6 words. Grammatical structure was appropriate. Vocabulary and language comprehension measures were above age level. Verbal retention span remained below age level.

Discussion. This child worked diligently the entire 16 months. She was supported by most understanding parents. In addition, she was involved in decision-making whenever and wherever possible (such as deciding among several reinforcements), and she was continually praised for her hard work. There were a few days she would not work, and she was allowed to play freely and talk about the frustrations and difficulty of the training. This was a rare occurrence however.

An unexpected but very important outcome of the training program was the gradual shift of responsibility for altering the signal dimensions from the clinician to the child. That is, the processes of prolonging the signal, reducing the presentation rate, and increasing the repetitions employed by the clinician to facilitate signal detection were slowly incorporated by the child as her own strategy for identification. It became automatic for her to prolong and repeat the signal aloud to herself when she was unsure of the correct identification. In addition, she developed strategies that used other modalities to help her. For example, an audible repetition of a word was accompanied by both vocal and motoric emphasis on the target phoneme. To identify the position of the sound in the word, she moved her finger across space left to right as through visualizing the phonetic sequence.

The "place" discrimination training was a very significant component of building the phonetic structure into perception. The need to search through the word for the position of the target sound related the specific phonemes to the variety of phonetic contexts in which they might occur. In this way, the child learned to extract only the relevant information within the context, and also to experience the effect of context on the target sounds.

Several other factors that seemed to contribute to the success of the program and the motivation of the child were (1) using a review and warm-up period prior to each session; (2) organizing trials in blocks of ten with short breaks in between and representing these graphically to the child; (3) maintaining a high success rate; (4) programming in very small increments of difficulty; (5) giving the child very clear directions and warning her when a change in signal was made; and (6) continually monitoring both the quantitative and qualitative aspects of the child's performance as a guide to programming.

Summary. In summary, the experience with this child suggests (1) that an auditory processing disability of some kind did exist and was responsive to treatment; (2) that improvement in auditory processing was associated with improvement in speech and language; and (3) that some degree of auditory disability persisted but was controlled by the child by using various strategies to facilitate identification of the auditory signal.

Addendum. This child has been followed through three years of school. She continues to present with normal speech and language behavior. She does average or above in school. Reading comprehension scores are at grade level while word recognition skills are somewhat below grade level.

CONCLUSION

Auditory processing disorders in children can be identified through careful evaluation using a full battery of speech and language tests and several informal measures of sound discrimination. The pattern of scores and the qualitative aspects of the child's responses will provide the evidence for identification. It is possible to treat these disorders with a systematic program of perceptual training in those cues and contrasts important to the accurate reception of speech. This kind of training results in the general improvement of language as well. Only through more and more careful and precise evaluation and treatment methods can we begin to understand the nature of this disorder further, and coroborate the findings of further research.

REFERENCES

1. Kirk SA, McCarthy JJ, Kirk WD: Illinois Test of Psycholinguistic Abilities, Revised. Urbana, University of Illinois Press, 1975
2. Baker HJ, Leland B: Detroit Tests of Learning Aptitude. Indianapolis, Bobbs-Merrill, 1935, revised 1959
3. Dunn LM: Peabody Picture Vocabulary Test. Circle Pines, Minnesota, American Guidance Service, 1959
4. Carrow E: Test for Auditory Comprehension of Language. Boston, Teaching Resources, 1973
5. Dunn LM, Markwardt FC Jr: Peabody Individual Achievement Test. Circle Pines, Minnesota, American Guidance Service, 1970
6. Carrow E: Carrow Elicited Language Inventory. Boston, Teaching Resources, 1974

7. Tallal P, Stark R, Curtiss B: The relation between speech perception impairment and speech production impairment in children with developmental dysphasia. Brain Lang 3:305–317, 1976
8. Wepman J: Wepman Test of Auditory Discrimination. Chicago, Language Research Associates, 1973
9. Goldman R, Fristoe M, Woodcock RW: Goldman-Fristoe-Woodcock Auditory Skills Test Battery. Circle Pines, Minnesota, American Guidance Service, 1974
10. Harris C: Auditory processing disability: Sixteen months of treatment, in Andrews JR, Burns MS (eds): Selected Papers in Language and Phonology, vol II. Evanston, Institute for Continuing Professional Education, 1977, pp 1–6
11. Tallal P, Piercy M: Defects of non-verbal auditory perception in children with developmental aphasia. Nature 241:468–469, 1973
12. Tallal P, Piercy M: Developmental aphasia: Impaired rate of non-verbal processing as a function of sensory modality. Neuropsychologia 11:389–398, 1973
13. Tallal P, Piercy M: Developmental aphasia: Rate of auditory processing and selective impairment of consonant perception. Neuropsychologia 12:83–94, 1974
14. Tallal P, Piercy M: Developmental aphasia: The perception of brief vowels and extended stop consonants. Neuropsychologia 13:69–74, 1975
15. Tallal P: Perceptual and linguistic factors in the language impairment of developmental aphasics: An experimental investigation with the Token Test. Cortex 11:196–205, 1975

Kathleen L. Johnston

8

Auditory Processing in Aphasic Adults: Relationship between Language Disorders and Auditory Processing Disorders

The words; there is something very wrong. Not wrong, exactly, but not right, either. Cockeyed–it is cockeyed. Like a big–(gestures to indicate a wide expanse of considerable depth). You see the one you want and reach for it. What comes out is very wrong. You see the one again and reach for it and what comes out is wrong. Then you–everything goes cockeyed. You don't know, you can't tell–.

Someone, somewhere must know what to do. You see, it isn't hard. It isn't wrong–just cockeyed. Just a little–twisted. Someone must know how to fix it up. It isn't hard.

Aphasic Patient, 2-6-68

The patient who spoke these words has an auditory processing disorder in conjunction with aphasia. His description of what happens during his search for words is excellent. He presents the image of a large repository of words stored in his brain; he knows they are there because he can "see" them. At least, in some sense, there is awareness of the individual presence of words. He goes through some undefined searching process and is able to select a desired word. But somewhere between the pool of words in his brain and his mouth, something goes awry. The word that is spoken is not the word selected. The word used may be related to the anticipated word by meaning, or it may sound very similar to it. He recognizes the word spoken as incorrect, and he undertakes the searching process again. The desired word is found, but again, when spoken, it is not the same one he believed he would say. Then, as he becomes concerned about this process, something happens which seems to erase all that he knew before. He can't find the word in the repository, or if he does find it, he is no longer certain that it is the one he was looking for.

This patient's unexpected eloquence stems from his firm belief that there is only some little thing that is wrong. He believes that it will take only a very small adjustment to make it better. In the end, he is pleading for understanding. He is saying that you are making it more difficult than it needs to be. But, in fact, sometimes it is extremely difficult to resolve his problem because the nature of auditory processing and its relationship to language processing is not fully understood. The aphasic problem becomes confused with the auditory processing disorder, and traditional aphasia therapy methods are not always sufficient to stimulate language recovery. Auditory processing disorders are frequently treated inadequately and the patient is discharged from therapy without having made maximal progress.

There are several different kinds of auditory processing disorders that appear with aphasia. The purpose of this chapter is to discuss these processes, their identification and measurement using traditional aphasia test batteries, and their relationship to language processing. This discussion provides a framework in which auditory processing and language disturbance can be considered. The final aim is to specify how an understanding of these auditory disorders can facilitate rehabilitation.

APHASIA

Aphasia is a disorder of language. Patients with aphasia have difficulty retrieving the learned language code. This results in a reduction of vocabulary whether the patient is listening, speaking, reading, or writing. Other associated symptoms include reduction of verbal retention span, disturbances in sound production, and impaired perception of the speech signal. The loss of language perception is not due to lack of hearing acuity but to misinterpretation of the speech signals. Most adult aphasic patients have some impairment in the auditory processing of language. This is the result of dysfunction at the cerebral level of the auditory system.

Observation, analysis, and measurement of the response patterns of aphasic patients have given rise to a multitude of classification systems that sometimes clarify and sometimes confuse our understanding of aphasic symptomatology. For example, Macmahon[1] has identified 113 words used in the literature to identify types of aphasia; some are synonymous, and others are not necessarily mutually exclusive. Some terms reflect the anatomic location of the lesion causing the symptomatology; others reflect the name of a predominant symptom that occurs as a result of the lesion.

Patients who suffer lesions in the anterior cerebral cortex (see Fig. 8-1) are noted to have similar symptomatology.[2] Patients with anterior aphasia (also called Broca's aphasia, motor aphasia, expressive aphasia, and nonfluent aphasia) have, as their most predominant symptom, difficulty in expressing speech. They have awkward articulation, limited vocabulary, and restriction of grammar to the simplest, most overlearned forms.[3] Historically, patients with anterior lesions were not believed to have much, if any, difficulty with auditory comprehension.

Patients who suffer lesions in the posterior cerebral cortex (see Fig. 8-1) exhibit symptoms that are quite different from those with anterior lesions. In posterior aphasia (also called Wernicke's aphasia, sensory aphasia, receptive aphasia, and fluent aphasia), the most predominant symptom is difficulty with comprehension. This is due to a variety of auditory processing difficulties. Patients have speech that is fluent, but frequently quite meaningless. The patient might simply repeat the words he hears or express sound combinations meaningless to the language (jargon). More mildly involved patients have well-articulated speech that contains misplaced or extraneous sounds (paraphasias).[3]

Other terms used for classification of aphasia attempt to differentiate the varying degrees of severity present and the kind of involvement of the auditory system. Some of the terms used to describe patients who exhibit jargon are jargon aphasia, aphasia with intermittent auditory imperception, Wernicke's aphasia, sensory aphasia, acoustic-gnostic aphasia, and syntactical aphasia.

Terms used to classify aphasia in which jargon is not present, but in which various kinds of auditory processing disorders exist are conduction or central aphasia, transcortical sensory aphasia, anomic aphasia, and pure word deafness. These terms are applied to patients according to the degree of difficulty found in repetition, in comprehension, and in word finding.

Sometimes these classifications are lumped together under the more general terms of posterior aphasia, receptive aphasia, fluent aphasia, or Wernicke's aphasia. It is generally agreed that lesions producing the posterior aphasias involve the posterior temporal or the posterior temporoparietal region of the major hemisphere.[4] Figure 8-1 and Table 8-1 show the cortical areas of involvement for aphasia, and the six most common and universally recognized aphasic syndromes related to them.

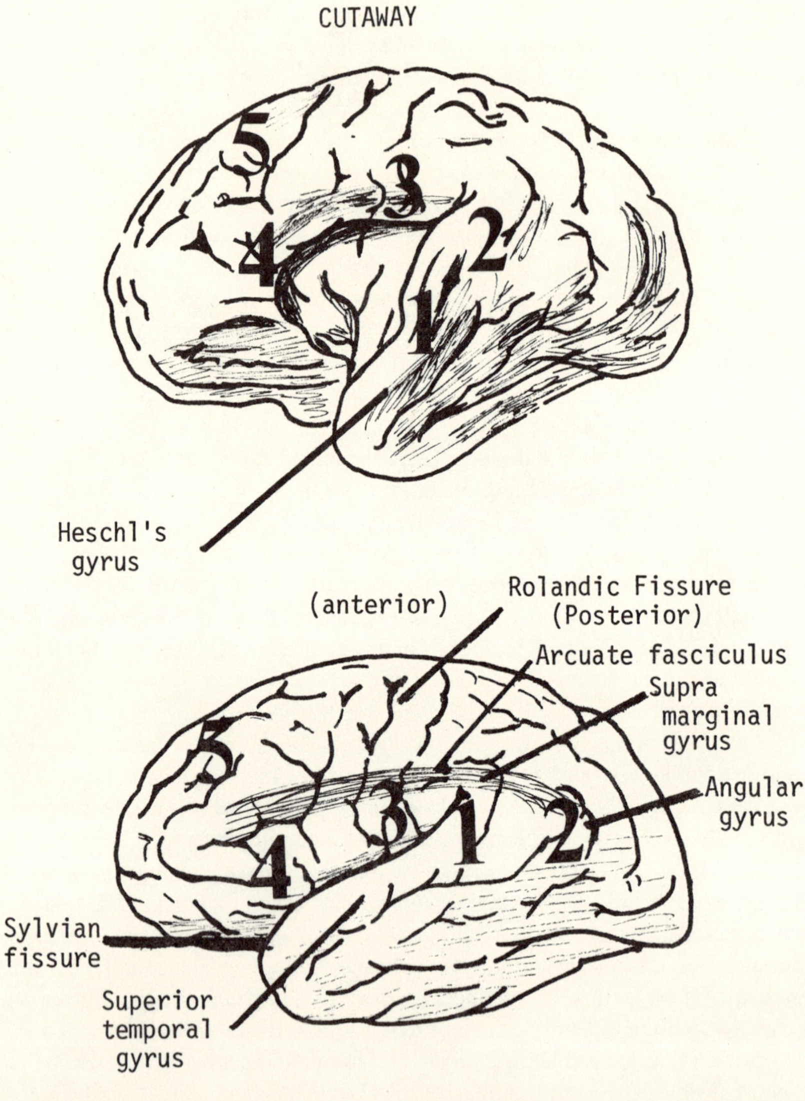

Fig. 8-1. Lateral aspect of the brain (left hemisphere).

Table 8-1
Aphasic Syndromes and Their Related Location of Lesion as Determined by Brain Scanning*

1. *Wernicke's aphasia:* Auditory comprehension is impaired. Speech is fluently articulated, but paraphasic. (Possible involvement 2, 3)
2. *Anomia:* Prominence of word finding difficulty in the context of fluent, grammatically well-formed speech. Literal and verbal paraphasias are absent. Auditory comprehension is relatively intact. (Remote brain)
3. *Conduction aphasia:* Auditory comprehension is near normal, repetition is severely impaired as compared to fluencey level in spontaneous speech. Many literal paraphasias in spontaneous speech. (Possible involvement 1, 2)
4. *Broca's aphasia:* Auditory comprehension relatively preserved. Articulation is awkward, vocabulary is limited and grammar is restricted to the simplest, most overlearned forms. (Possible involvement, none)
5. *Transcortical motor aphasia:* Auditory comprehension is relatively well spared, repetition is intact. Spontaneous speech is relatively limited. (Possible involvement, none)
6. *Global aphasia:* Auditory comprehension is severely limited, as is speech production (speech consists only of automatic speech). Patient is unable to name or repeat. (Possible involvement 2, 3)

Reprinted from Heilman K: Neuropsychologic changes in the stroke patient. Geriatrics 29:153–160, 1974 with permission.

*The number preceeding the definition identifies the area of involvement in Figure 8-1. The numbers following the definitions relate to areas of possible involvement, depicted in Figure 8-1.

Researchers have attempted to isolate and identify each of these aphasic groups by symptomatology and by locus of lesion. There is good evidence in the literature to indicate that the variation of symptomatology observed in aphasia can be explained, in part, by the variation in location of the lesion as determined by brain scanning.[5, 6] However, this kind of research needs to incorporate a more comprehensive and detailed examination of aphasic behavior before direct correlations between site of lesion and aphasic symptomatology can be made. The size, extent, and location of the cortical lesions found on studies correlating language deficit with brain scanning do not entirely account for individual differences in the kind and degree of language disturbance found in aphasic patients.[6]

Patient symptomatology does not fall easily into one or the other of these recognized classification groups. Sometimes this is because the lesions responsible for the aphasia are large and result in mixed varieties.[7] Head[8] states that any organic process that gravely impairs speech also disturbs other functions not usually classified with language, and spares and leaves unaffected much that undoubtedly belongs to it. The more carefully a patient is examined the less certain one is that his disorder corresponds with any preconceived category. Macmahon,[1] who offers an interesting commentary on the state of chaos which exists in the use of terminology, suggests that another cause of the problem of classification is that aphasia has traditionally been classified by neurologists who are specialized in anatomic structure, rather than by linguists who are specialized in language.

Current terminology does not reflect the wide range of knowledge gained by research presenting strong evidence that the classical division of anterior and posterior aphasias does not reflect the facts about language. Studies support the idea that disorders of the language system in aphasic patients are similar regardless of the location of the lesion. For example, Blumstein *et al.*[9] found that Wernicke's aphasics were not the most impaired on a task of phoneme (sound) discrimination. They believed that the results of their study indicated that a disturbance of phonemic hearing is not limited to temporal lobe patients but is found in varying degrees in all the aphasic groups tested. In another study,[10] Blumstein concluded that patients having anterior and posterior pathology exhibited similar errors in ordering phonemic sequences.

Goodglass[11] investigated inflectional endings and determined that all aphasic patients performed similarly regardless of their clinical groupings. In another study,[12] he found no evidence that particular grammatical rules were harder for agrammatic aphasics than for fluent aphasics. Gardner, Denes, and Zurif[13] devised a sentence reading test in order to assess aphasic patients' ability to detect errors in written discourse. They found no difference in overall scores between patients with anterior and posterior pathology. They did find that anterior patients performed somewhat better on the oral version of the test, while posterior patients did better on the written version of the test. They concluded that reading for meaning is a relatively uniform process in aphasia.[13]

AUDITORY PROCESSING

The language system and the auditory system maintain an intricate relationship.[14] Although language processing exists independent of the auditory system (as seen in the congenitally deaf), it appears that normal language development and the development of speech are dependent upon an intact auditory system. Research on the acoustic properties of speech sounds, investigations of dichotic listening, and the linguistic analysis of language have contributed much in the past two decades to our understanding of central processing. Yet neither the scope nor the complexity of the activities taking place in these two systems are fully understood.[15]

For some patients, auditory processing disorders are not just secondary complications that appear with the language disturbance, but are a primary disorder. In these cases, traditional aphasia therapy techniques are frequently ineffectual. Although mechanisms underlying auditory disturbances may remain elusive to the therapist, some attempt to delineate among processing components can make a startling difference in the methods of rehabilitation that are chosen. Problems of differential diagnosis in aphasia occur most frequently in patients with auditory impairment, and they can be minimized by this kind of awareness on the part of the clinician. A brief review of the auditory system and a summary of how it operates will underscore the complexity of the task at hand, and will identify the focus for the paradigm which follows.

Auditory System

The auditory system includes the ear, the eighth cranial nerve, the brain stem, and the cerebral cortex—more specifically, the temporal lobes of the cortex. The primary auditory receiving areas (Heschl's gyri) are situated in the temporal lobes of the right and left hemispheres (Fig. 8-1). Each area receives inpute from both ears, but has no intelligent recognition of sounds. The left primary receiving area has a more direct pathway to the language areas which are located in the left (or dominant) hemisphere.[16]

Specialized neurons in Heschl's gyri act primarily as a relay station: they receive input from each ear and transmit it to other specialized neurons. These neurons, located in Wernicke's area, translate sounds into language symbols. They exist only in one cerebral hemisphere, the dominant hemisphere for speech, which for most individuals is the left hemisphere.[16]

The right auditory receiving area appears to be specialized for processing environmental sounds (car starting, water running), nonverbal products of the vocal tract (coughing, humming), and Gestalt perception (environmental sounds not requiring linguistic analysis).[16] The left auditory receiving area appears to be specialized for processing the speech signal and also its components.[17, 18] There is strong evidence, however, that normally both hemispheres are actively engaged in the processing of both verbal and nonverbal acoustic stimuli.[19, 21] The right nondominant hemisphere appears to be equipped to process some auditory-verbal stimuli.[22-24] The right hemisphere appears to comprehend normal context dependent connected discourse and to be able to initiate a limited amount of propositional speech. It apparently is less well equipped to process complex linguistic messages with multiple references or to initiate functional speech.[25, 26]

The central process which combines speech information from the two ears may operate in an additive manner. Cullen *et al.*[27] suggest that the information handling capacity for this process is slightly greater than the capacity for a single ear and that, before central combination, speech information carried by one ear is independent of speech information carried by the other. They note that additional neural relays may be required to transmit information from the right primary auditory cortex to the left temporal parietal cortex for final processing.

Auditory Processing Paradigm: A Compilation of Ideas

The auditory processing paradigm that follows incorporates ideas taken from the literature, from the author's experience, and, hopefully, from common sense. It is not definitive, but it does offer a schematic way of isolating and integrating some of the probable component parts of this highly complex and vital central process.

Auditory processing begins with the perception of the acoustic signal and includes the classification of the signal as language rather than simply noise. Once the signal is perceived, an analysis of (phonologic) linguistic units which combine to form words takes place. The listener must *attend* to each incoming signal, *analyze* all signal units, and *store* what he has perceived into short term memory. Next, the listener must *judge* which signal units are pertinent to his purpose, and *retain* that information in long term memory. Here it is processed again, syntactically and semantically, for meaning. He may also process it phonologically into motor patterns necessary for articulation. Meaning is abstracted from the incoming signal by a complex series of phonetic, morphologic and semantic *associations*.

Table 8-2 delineates these processes in more detail.

Table 8-2
Auditory Processing Paradigm

Listener must:

1. Attend to each incoming signal.[28] On a prelinguistic level, attention includes the perception of an acoustic signal and an awareness that the sound has meaning.
   A. Noise: environmental sounds not requiring linguistic analysis which appear to be processed in the right auditory receiving area (Heschl's gyrus).[16]
   B. Speech/language: differentiated from noise on the basis of the reception of different component phonetic elements, singly or in combination.[29]
2. Analyze all signal units.[30]
   A. Acoustics: analyzing the vibratory form of energy that produces sound.[31] The "pure tone" is a simple sinusoidal acoustic signal defined by frequency and intensity. Complex tones depend also upon phase relations (time relations) among the component pure tones. Speech is made up of varied complex tones.[32]
   B. Phonetics: related to acoustics and physiology.[30] Phonetic elements are the shortest units of speech that can be recognized as having stable identity:

Table 8-2 (continued)

vowels (pure tones of distinctive pattern), diphthongs, and consonants. Phonetics is also concerned with the combinations of these simple sounds: syllables, words, and connected phrases.[33]

C. Phonemics: concerned with the analysis of the speech signal from a linguistic point of view.[34] It is the study of the units which make up language, and of the rules for sequencing and combining these units for the expression of thought.

3. Store into short-term memory.[30]
   A. Auditory memory: the memory store in which an uncategorized, image-like representation of an auditory stimulus is briefly held after presentation. It is the memory store which precedes short term memory.[35]
   B. Short term memory (audioverbal memory): refers to the holding for preliminary analysis and categorization of sounds, syllables, and words.[36, 37] It appears to facilitate some aspects of language processing,[38] and some aspects of language processing seem to facilitate it.[39]
4. Select the signal units which are appropriate to the purpose.
   A. Matching to previously stored patterns: if the pattern that is forming is familiar, the analysis can proceed to the next signal.
   B. Meaning: a verbal label is attached to the signal unit.[16, 36]
   C. Coding: the signal units are coded with respect to different rules.[28, 30, 36]
      1. Syntactic: rules for combining words into phrases, clauses, and sentences.
      2. Semantic: rules which govern the categorization of the meaning of words.
      3. Phonologic: (perhaps this is included here) signals are processed into motor patterns necessary for articulation.
      4. Associational: meaning is abstracted from the incoming signals by a complex series of phonetic, morphologic, and semantic associations.[16]
5. Retain the information in long term memory[28, 30] Long term memory is less sensitive to retention time than is short term memory but is dependent upon variables such as rate of presentation, word frequency, and opportunity for rehearsal.[40] Memory is a byproduct of the extent to which an individual analyzes the verbal information during the time it is presented. The more distinctive features the individual can analyze, the greater the probability of eventual retrieval.[41]

Language

The auditory processes described above would have to link up with the language system on many levels. Language involves many additional steps, perhaps beginning with the formation of an idea. Vocabulary selection and arrangement of words in a suitable semantic and syntactic framework would also be included. Finally, a complete description of language use would have to encompass the skilled motor movements (speech) that are the means of expression.

Understanding how auditory processing and language processing work together is difficult. The comprehension of language obviously requires the interaction of both processes. According to the auditory processing paradigm, comprehension may be initiated earlier, but it is developed and completed in Steps 4 and 5. Pick[29] offers a list of possible steps for the comprehension of language which begin after phonemes are correctly identified:

1. A word is heard correctly and can be repeated automatically but is not understood.
2. A word is heard correctly and can be repeated deliberately but is not understood.
3. Understanding of the word comes with repetition of the word and/or other cueing.
4. The word evokes other concepts related in content which allow correct understanding.
5. The word is understood without difficulty.
6. The sentence is understood.

Comprehension is apparently related to just how much of the signal the patient is able to analyze, and how much he is able to remember. Repetition of the signals or other cueing offers the aphasic patient more opportunity to extract distinctive phonemic, semantic, and conceptual features for analysis. Comprehension appears to be multidimensional, and probably evolves through the operations of several different processes. Although lack of comprehension can occur at the phonemic level, there is evidence that noncomprehension is also likely to occur at the semantic level. Coughland and Warrington[42] suggest that word comprehension and word retrieval impairments found in patients with left hemisphere lesions reflect deficits in semantic memory.

In reviewing this background information it becomes evident that there is confusion regarding the use of terminology, perplexity about the classical anterior and posterior division, and doubts concerning auditory and language processing and their relationships. However, these questions are being answered, and new terminology based on increased knowledge will reflect more precise descriptions of patient behavior.

EVALUATING THE APHASIC PATIENT

Before discussing some of the more formalized aphasia test batteries in relationship to auditory processing, several comments about language and patients with language disorders must be made. It is important to remember that language does not consist solely of the more formalized behavior so far discussed. Nonverbal behavior (tone of voice, gesture, posture, body movements, spatial orientation, physical proximity, eye contact, facial expression) is capable of conveying considerable information.[43] Patients with impaired ability to use language usually have not lost their ability to use or comprehend these features of communication. A patient whose language is severely impaired is sometimes able to perform paralinguistic tasks well enough to deceive friends and family into believing the language deficit is not as severe as they have been led to believe. Davis Howes[44] distinguishes between language and appreciation of meaning:

> Chimpanzees and other higher apes cannot acquire speech, although they possess both vocal skills and learning capacity of high order and appear to appreciate the meaning of events and situations, except for their lack of language,* much as we do. Aphasic patients exhibit a clear loss of capability for language and for learning verbal (but not nonverbal) materials, but they do retain their appreciation of meanings along with the capacity for expressing them without the use of words. [p. 181]

The distinction between language capability and appreciation of meaning is not always easily made when working with severely involved patients. Consider the following description of patient behavior:

> She tried diligently to perform on the aphasia test battery. She listened intently while the examiner named pictures. She understood that she was to point to the one named. She pleaded with her eyes and with gestures for multiple repetitions of the word. Her hand would reach out toward a picture—incorrect—and then she would withdraw it, shaking her head. She could not follow directions, not point to colors, numbers, or letters. She could not verbalize; she could not point to any object or picture correctly; she could not match written words to pictures; she could not read sentences and paragraphs; she could not write anything either to dictation or spontaneously. She did not perform one test item correctly, yet she patiently tried to respond. She exhibited a severe aphasia, and her behavior indicated a severe auditory processing disorder as well. When the examiner got up to leave, she looked the woman carefully in the eye and said, "You are wearing the most beautiful ring I have ever seen." The woman smiled, held out her hand, removed her ring and offered it to the examiner for inspection.**

This patient clearly appreciates meaning but, in addition, she has a language system that is working, although severely impaired. She gives two important, although not infallible, clues that she can make considerable recovery in language. The first is that she tried to perform on the test battery, indicating her sustained belief that she could perform some task. The second

*Recently, experiments with apes reveal that they can learn language. Howes apparently is referring to behavior in their native setting.

**Taken from personal files.

is that she responded correctly to a personal directive that was not accompanied by visual cues. The latter can be explained only hypothetically: perhaps the rigors of formal testing overload a system that can function imperfectly in an informal and personal situation.

This patient is not to be confused with the patient classified as having global aphasia in which brain damage involves both Wernicke's and Broca's areas and their connecting pathways. Global aphasia results in very limited comprehension, nonfluent speech that consist of overlearned terms (that's for sure', 'damn right'), and automatic speech (counting, saying the days of the week). Patients with global aphasia have extensive brain damage and do not regain language function, although some may respond to personal directives when accompanied by visual cues.

Schuell and Johnston[45] found that over two-thirds of the patients tested soon after onset, and classified as having global aphasia, were reclassified three months later as having either Broca's aphasia, or aphasia with intermittent auditory imperception. Since thereapy recommendations are sometimes made on the basis of testing done when a patient is not stable, it is important to devise methods for separating these three patient groups on bases other than test scores alone.

The patient described in the example above exhibited a severe aphasia, complicated by additional involvement of the auditory processes—involvement more extensive than is seen in aphasia alone. Patients having these symptoms can improve with the aid of therapy, and it is important to differentiate them from those having global aphasia. Aphasia test scores are not particularly helpful in identifying these patients. However, when the clinician looks for patterns in the patient's performance and interprets these in the light of theories of auditory processing, he may be able to pinpoint the primary processing disorders.

Aphasia Test Batteries

Traditional aphasia test batteries are general tests of language performance. They are compromises between the quick, bedside examination the neurologists prefer, and the more complete delineation of performance (or lack of performance) that speech and language therapists require. They offer the clinician a means of recording pertinent observations, and only imperfectly allow a means for analysis of these observations. Diagnostic batteries, such as the *Minnesota Test for the Differential Diagnosis of Aphasia* (MTDDA),[46] the *Boston Diagnostic Aphasia Examination* (BDAE),[3] the *Porch Index of Communicative Ability* (PICA),[47] and the *Neurosensory Center Comprehensive Examination for Aphasia* (NCCEA)[48] are excellent for the purposes for which they were intended. Administration time is such that testing can usually be accomplished at one sitting and materials may be administered at bedside.

Test results provide diagnostic information that enables the therapist to differentiate among various kinds of aphasia. This information is usually sufficient to enable a prognosis of the recovery of language function to be made to family and hospital staff, and to direct the clinician to a particular therapy goal.

An experienced examiner can make good use of an aphasia test battery for differential diagnosis of aphasia, and for clues regarding auditory processing disorders. Auditory discrimination errors are revealed by errors on tasks such as pointing to randomly named letters of the alphabet and discrimination between paired words. Patients with auditory processing disorders tend to confuse letters and words which have names that sound alike. Reduction of auditory retention span is revealed by the patients' performance on simple or complex commands, and by their ability to repeat digits, a word series and sentences. Patients who have a persistent auditory processing disorder make more errors on auditory tasks than do other patients. They frequently respond like global aphasic patients do on these subtests. For example, Schuell[49] found that only patients classified as having global aphasia or aphasia with intermittent auditory imperception made four errors or more on the task of discriminating between paired words. Patients not classified in these two groups made fewer errors.

Aphasia test batteries allow clinicians to make *inferences* about language and auditory processing. The quantitative results of testing are not always sufficient for differentiating minor but consistent patterns within aphasia classifications. Yet, it is the recognition of these patterns that enables the clinician to design a therapy program which will work effectively. Schuell[49] notes that a score informs only that a patient did or did not, for example, write a word to dictation. The score does not inform the examiner whether the patient *can* perform, but, assuming that the patient has performed to the best of his ability, it does suggest *where* the language breakdown occurs. In addition, we need to know *why* the breakdown occurs. Schuell points out further that, if the patient cannot write a word to dictation (assuming adequate muscular control), it could be for one or more of several reasons: he may have lost the names of the letters; he may have lost the letter sequence; he may not have "heard" the word; or he may not remember the word.[49]

Aphasia test batteries usually include tests for disturbances in auditory processing such as:

1. Tests of recognition of letters of the alphabet, of words, of phrases or of sentences.
2. Tests of discrimination between words that sound alike.
3. Tests of sequencing (judgments of temporal order).
4. Tests of comprehension.
5. Tests of auditory retention span.

These kinds of tests relate only generally to the auditory processing paradigm. Tests results usually identify problems patients have with the composite of auditory processes rather than with the individual elements which make up the whole. Consequently, most test batteries measure the patients' *secondary* language disturbance. That is, they measure a sampling of performance on auditory tasks that may not provide sufficient information to design therapy techniques for the rehabilitation of specific, *primary* functions of auditory processing. For example, scores on tests of discrimination do not of themselves indicate the reason for the difficulty which may occur at any point in the analysis of the signal (as shown in the paradigm), e.g. in sequencing, in combining, or in storing signal units. One method for the refinement of classification techniques is to offer additional testing to patients whose aphasia seems difficult to categorize. Some of these supplemental tests include the *Token Test*,[50] standardized vocabulary and reading tests, tests of phoneme discrimination, and a variety of others that are not necessarily related to auditory processing but can isolate specific problems patients may not otherwise reveal.

Psycholinguistic Approach

The examination of psycholinguistic variables is useful when attempting to identify specific processing problems in aphasia.[51] The rationale for using psycholinguistic principles is two-fold: (1) studies suggest that the organization of speech may be based on distinctive feature relations held among phonemes;[17] and (2) the study of linguistics offers a well-defined and accepted framework for classifying observations of language behavior for analysis of the behavior, and for measurement of the extent to which the behavior deviates from the norm.

A *distinctive feature* is the smallest meaningful differentiation between sounds of a language. For example, in the classification system presented in Table 8-3, /n/ and /m/ differ from one another by one distinctive feature—place of articulation. There is no universally accepted distinctive feature system used by linguists to differentiate how alike or how different two sounds are from one another. Authors tend to use articulatory features, the most common of which are place and manner of articulation. For example, in Table 8-3, /p/ and /f/ differ from one another by two distinctive features—one of place, and one of manner. Another feature system might ignore the frication feature and note that /p/ and /f/ differ from one another by one distinctive feature, place.[12] While the system offered here is useful in evaluating patterns in patient responses and in designing therapy techniques, it does pose some problems of comparison when other systems are used. For example, note that /w/, usually classified as bilabial, is classified as a velar place of articulation.

Table 8-3
Chart of English Consonants

Place of Articulation	Manner of Articulation								
	Stops		Fricatives		Affricates		Nasals	Lateral	Glides
	Voiceless	Voiced	Voiceless	Voiced	Voiceless	Voiced			
Bilabial	p	b					m		
Labiodental			f	v					
Dental									
Alveolar	t	d	s	z			n	l	r
Palatal			š	ž	č	ǰ			y
Velar	k	g					ŋ		w
Glottal			h						

Most aphasic patients' responses show perceptual confusions which differ minimally from the target word, and occur in a predictable fashion with regard to a distinctive feature model. Therapy based on feature contrasts with much opportunity for practice and with visual cueing, usually works quickly and effectively. Patients with auditory processing disorders and aphasia make more total errors of perception and more errors that are greater than single-feature differences, than do patients in other diagnostic groups.[52] Therapy for these patients is discussed in a subsequent chapter.

Describing the speech of a patient in terms of the number and kind of *paraphasias* used is another attempt to measure primary disturbances by noting psycholinguistic variables. There are various kinds of paraphasias discussed in the literature but the most common are verbal and literal paraphasias.[46, 53] A verbal paraphasia is the substitution of one correct word or phrase for another. These could be related semantically (cat/dog), auditorially (view/few), visually (horse/house), or not at all (gate/fire). A literal or phonemic paraphasia is the replacement or transposition of one or more sounds in otherwise correct words (Methipal Episcodist/Methodist Episcopal).

Goodglass and Kaplan[3] define a third kind of paraphasia, neologistic distortion, as the introduction of extraneous phonemes or the transposition of intended phonemes that occurs such that less than half of the intended word is discernible. In the extreme, distortions may take the form of neologistic jargon.

Buckingham and Kertesz[54] list six kinds of paraphasias:

1. A switch in only one distinctive feature (e.g., voice, bat/pat).
2. An anticipatory paraphasia in which phonemes are produced that occur later in the word or phrase (e.g., frayed sleeves/freed slaves).
3. A sequential paraphasia in which an anticipated phoneme is added to the original sequence rather than substituted (e.g., linloleum/linoleum).
4. The addition of a phoneme from the preceding utterance (e.g., November/Desvember).
5. A verbal substitution (e.g., a banana is a tropical suit).
6. A semantic substitution (e.g., kitchen chair/easy chair).

Patients with auditory processing disorders in addition to the aphasia continue to make literal paraphasic errors throughout the recovery period, particularly under conditions of stress. The number of literal paraphasias, and their persistence during the recovery period, indicates problems of auditory processing.

The study of paraphasias has not been extensive. There is more to learn before the analysis of paraphasias can be used as a conclusive tool for differential diagnosis. Beyn and Vlasenko[55] point out that verbal paraphasias have been studied without taking into account the grammatical parts of speech. Testing does differentiate between naming an object, for example, and naming actions. But in the interpretation of test scores, the significance of a normal performance on the former (objects), and no performance on the latter (actions), is not considered. Goodglass and associates[56] note that the order of difficulty between semantic categories is not usually considered in analyzing paraphasias even though it does exist and does change in relation to the kind of task the patient is performing, for example, comprehension or naming.

Analyzing patient responses in terms of distinctive features and paraphasias expand the sample of behavior that is observable for diagnoses and therapy planning. In addition, this data can promote a better understanding of the relationship between auditory and language processing.

Repetition Behavior

Describing the speech of a patient on repetition tasks is another attempt to measure the primary disturbances of language. We are, however, only beginning to understand how to analyze repetition responses and how to construct phrases and sentences that may differentiate groups of patients on a linguistic basis. Repetition is not a special function of language, but simply a method we use for testing patients.[57] Performance on repetition tasks provides a means of differentiation among aphasia classifications, and can provide an important clue to the type of auditory processing disorder a patient experiences. For example, depending upon the severity and type of aphasia, patients may:

1. Repeat words but not phrases or sentences.
2. Repeat phrases and sentences but not words.
3. Repeat with comprehension.
4. Repeat without comprehension.
5. Repeat the beginnings, but not the middles and endings of phrases or sentences.
6. Repeat the middles, but not the beginnings or endings of phrases or sentences.
7. Repeat the endings, but not the beginnings or middles of phrases or sentences.
8. Repeat the beginnings and the endings, but not the middle of phrases or sentences.
9. Repeat incorrectly, but paraphrase adequately.
10. Repeat intelligibly, but with paraphasic errors.

To further confuse things, there are patients who respond with different permutations of the points listed.

The identification of paraphasias, of errors of repetition, and of distinctive feature patterns are relatively meaningless unless considered within some framework of knowledge of the processes that may be disturbed. The evaluation and differential diagnosis of the aphasic patient depends on this kind of integration.

AUDITORY PROCESSING DISORDERS: SOME THEORETIC NOTIONS

Various theoretic notions have been proposed as the underlying mechanisms for auditory processing disorders. Some of these are described below.

The patient does not retain input long enough to complete the processing sequence.[49] Retention can be defined as remembering specific linguistic inputs over short or long periods of time.[58] It is one of the auditory processing functions that aphasia test batteries are designed to measure. Conclusions are drawn from the patient's performance on tasks like following commands or pointing to objects named in sequence. Inferences about retention also are made from the patient's responses on tasks like repeating phrases or sentences.

According to the auditory processing paradigm presented by this author, retention would fall under Step 3. Auditory retention of verbal messages is necessary before the auditory processing sequence can be completed.[14] Patients with retention problems may be able to repeat words, but not phrases or sentences. Or, they may be able to repeat the beginnings, but not the middles and endings, of phrases or sentences. For some reason, not thoroughly understood, patients with auditory retention problems typically retain the first, but not the last part of the message. This can be demonstrated by performance on testing and in therapy. There are, however, patients who have difficulty with auditory retention but do not fit into this pattern. Some patients remember only the final portion of the message. Others will paraphrase the message given, indicating retention of meaning but not retention of, perhaps, the phonemics of the language. In view of this it seems very probable that problems of auditory retention result from more than one auditory processing disorder. To speak in terms of a reduced auditory retention span can be descriptive of patient behavior, but it does not appear to be particularly precise. For a clearer understanding of auditory processing, the causes of the reduction of auditory retention span must be investigated. The following theoretic notions offer alternative explanations.

The patient needs more processing time to analyze the signal.[49] One reason for reduced auditory retention may be that the patient's auditory system is functioning at a reduced rate of speed so that more processing time is needed to analyze signals. Initial messages are decoded, but as messages keep coming, they jam the analyzing system and cause succeeding units to be lost and go unperceived. This is a very tenable theory, and it offers possible explanations for patient performance in light of the auditory processing paradigm. For example, if each analysis performed on a word or phrase takes a certain amount of time, and if analysis involves phonologic, syntactic, semantic and associational levels, then, a patient with an impaired auditory system may have too little time to perform all the necessary analyses; his system could break down at any point on any level. This could explain the variety of performances observed on repetition tasks, and it could explain the lack of appreciation of meaning of some signals.

It is known that some aphasic patients benefit from more processing time than the normal listener needs.[59] These patients make fewer errors when the rate of presentation of stimuli is slowed, and when the pauses between words are lengthened.[28] A factor which has not yet been thoroughly investigated is the possibility that slower rates might result in improved performance for isolated words, but that phrases and sentences are best perceived when a normal speaking rate is used.[60]

Processing time is a measurable auditory function, and some aphasia batteries consider it in the scoring of some tests. By keeping track of patients' delayed responses on a variety of tests, inferences may be drawn as to the situations in which patients begin to experience difficulty and could benefit from a reduced presentation rate. In therapy, a normal speaking rate usually offers the best results in conversational speech, but on some specific tasks, slowing the presentation rate can elicit correct responses where only failures existed.

The patient experiences defective timing or sequencing of the input signals. The presence of sequencing disorders can be noted by asking the patient to repeat a series of rhythmic taps in imitation of the examiner. Music and rhythm have been considered to be the sole province of the nondominant hemisphere,[4] but there is reason to believe that rhythmic auditory stimuli are mediated by the speech hemisphere.[4, 61] Patients with auditory processing disorders usually experience difficulty in recognizing the rhythmic pattern unless it is executed slowly. There are patients who may recognize the rhythm but be unable to perform when asked to carry it out in series. They tend to continue tapping until the examiner indicates they may stop. Some patients perceive no pattern, but perform the correct number of taps. Since patients with sequencing disorders may also exhibit disturbances of phonemic hearing, another way to note the presence of timing or sequencing disturbances is by noting the number of literal paraphasias in the patient's speech.

Patients experiencing this type of disorder may know the number of syllables in the word, or the number of words in the sentence, but not the pattern which enables them to formulate the word or sentence. They usually understand the approximate meaning of the stimulus and can paraphrase it adequately. Sometimes, even when provided with the printed sentence, the patient can not read the syllables or words in correct sequence.

Patients tend to have more difficulty on verbal sequencing tasks as the length and/or the complexity of the stimuli increases. Some patients are able to show pictorially or graphically the proper sequence while still unable to verbalize it. Often, patients are able to indicate awareness of their errors and even correct them, so long as they do not have to repeat the entire sequence. This behavior suggests that while sequencing disorders are disorders of auditory processing, they are less intricately related to the language system than other auditory disturbances under discussion.

Some patients having sequencing difficulties become impatient with having to repeat sentences because they believe it is a ridiculous exercise as long as they understand the meaning—which they often do not understand. One such patient, asked to repeat, 'I want a hamburger, a cup of coffee, and a malted milk', said, "I went to the drugstore and bought a malted milk. Oh, and a hamburger." After reading the sentence aloud, the patient pointed out that a drugstore was as good a place as any to buy a hamburger, and that he would not buy coffee anyway because he did not drink it. He saw no point in trying to repeat the sentence as it was given. Such patients become much more tractable when errors of comprehension and their relationship to proper sequencing are demonstrated to them.

The patient is unable to perceive the message. Perception of the input signal would certainly influence retention, since one cannot retain what has not been perceived. Isolation of a perceptual problem could be difficult since it might exist along any part of the message. The patient may have difficulty differentiating the classes of sounds (e.g., voiced/voiceless). This is not usually examined in language tests. He may have difficulty with the temporal features of sounds (e.g., /p/vs/s/). Or, he may have difficulty with pattern perception and recognition which is tested by discrimination between sound pairs.[62]

Tests of auditory discrimination sometimes included in language batteries offer the therapist some idea of the existence of a problem with perception. For example, the *MTDDA*[46] includes a task for discriminating between similar phonemes in common words. Other tests which require the patient to point to letters of the alphabet named by the examiner might serve a similar function.

Patients having difficulty with perception may perform better in the other modalities of language, such as reading or writing, but usually the perceptual problems are reflected in reading and writing performance as well. Examining errors made in a task such as writing letters to dictation might reveal sound class errors representative of the kinds of perceptual confusions the patient makes. If the perceptual problem is identified and a therapy plan utilizing visual reinforcement is devised, the patient can improve. Lack of improvement often means that the therapist has not isolated the perceptual problem and is working on stimuli too complex for the patient to analyze and absorb.

The patient exhibits a reduction of information resulting from defective matching with previously stored patterns.[49] It is possible that a complete analysis of frequently recurring and/or anticipated sounds or words may not be necessary. Instead, the familiar signal may be matched with previously stored patterns and, if recognized, further analysis may be terminated. Matching could occur on the sound level and on the more complex levels of syllables and words. Defective matching could occur if the patient incorrectly believed the signal matched a particular stored unit when it did not, or if he incorrectly believed it did not match when it did. For example, a patient might repeat a word and say, "Snow. Snow. Am I saying it right? Snow? It doesn't sound right. It doesn't mean anything. It is funny—I had this before and it sounded okay." Later, he might say, "Ohhhh, snow! Why didn't you say it that way before?" Another patient might repeat the word incorrectly and it will sound right to him. For example, with one patient several varying attempts were made to elicit the word, 'kitchen'. The patient kept repeating the word, 'chicken'. Finally he became irritated and said, "Sink. Water. Dish. I *know* it is chicken. Chicken, chicken, chicken. I *am* saying chicken!"

Of course, these examples might be equally illustrative of other auditory processing problems. Saying 'chicken' for 'kitchen' could be a perceptual problem or even a problem of sequencing. 'Snow' might illustrate a problem of comprehension. Defective matching might be the result of a more basic perceptual problem. This issue is not well resolved in the literature.

The patient exhibits a reduction of information resulting from impaired scanning processes. Normal listeners screen out background noises, attending primarily to the stimulus presented to them. They do not attend to every portion of the signal, but make predictions and assumptions of what is to come based on what they have already perceived. One patient became so involved with hearing every sound in every word that he was unable to grasp the meaning of words. It appears as though the inability to make predictions results in attention to every portion of the signal at the price of reduced comprehension. Scanning problems are not unique to the posterior aphasias but occur in anterior aphasias as well.

In some patients, background noise reduces perception. One patient became very upset in therapy and indicated that he heard a noise so bothersome that it prevent him from hearing the therapist. The therapist could perceive no sounds at the times the patient indicated they were present. Gradually, the therapist became aware that the patient was responding to the hospital paging system which was so faint that it was barely perceptible even with concentration. Other patients have experienced the same difficulty with background noise from lawnmowers, radios, and airplanes. One patient incorporated part of a conversation held behind closed doors in another room into his therapy response. This difficulty might represent a type of scanning problem. In every case, as the patient improved in language, the difficulties with background noises ceased.

The patient exhibits a reduction of information because of interference in the system.[49, 63] This hypothesis encompasses patients' complaints that signals seem garbled although there is no readily available external explanation for the type of interference they experience. Whatever the problem may be, it interferes with the perception of signals, and is ameliorated with the recovery of language function.

Scheull[49] recognized that noise (interference) in the auditory system prevented some patients from perceiving signals. Patients behaved as though they were working very hard to listen. They tired quickly and tended to make more errors at the end of the therapy session than at the beginning. They stated by words or gestures when they had had enough. One woman, after 20 minutes of therapy, would push the materials aside and say, "I can't listen anymore."

For some patients it appears as though the structure of the sentence is needed in order for appreciation of meaning to occur. For example, a patient was asked to repeat, 'I put butter on my potatoes'. He began, "I put butter . . .," and then he asked for a repetition of the stimulus. After several attempts, he still did not proceed beyond, "I put butter." The therapist asked, "Can you tell me in your own words, where *you* put butter?" The patient became confused and frustrated, and was unable to respond, although he continued to try to retrieve the original sentence. After he was able to repeat the original sentence, he was able to state that he put butter in the refrigerator or on the table.

Brookshire[63] discussed the notion of "noise build-up," and his description of patient behavior agrees with the previous example with one important exception—he found no evidence that these patients also had an inability to appreciate the meaning of the phrases and sentences. He identified a separate group of patients with "information capacity deficit," and he stated that the performance of these patients tends to be alternately good and poor within a given auditory message. He stated, "If these patients are asked to repeat a series of words or a sentence, they tend to report the first and last elements in the series or the sentence, and leave out, or make errors on the middle elements." [p. 80]

Defective matching, impaired scanning, and noise in the system affect the patient's perception of the signal. Now that psycholinguistics has offered a more systematic approach to the study of language than has been used previously, these approaches to the evaluation of perception hopefully will yield a more comprehensive understanding of these mechanisms.

The patient experiences a reduction of information from a weak and/or intermittent input signal.[64] These patients speak in jargon initially. They gradually add more correct sounds until speech becomes intelligible, even though it contains paraphasias. The auditory imperception seems to have an on-off effect. For example, patients respond correctly to test items or therapy materials for six to ten trials, then, suddenly, every response is incorrect. Some patients may, after responding correctly for ten items and missing the next eight, begin responding with answers which were required on the previous questions. It is almost as though the patient cut out, and then came to and continued where he left off, regardless of the immediate item. Harris[52] demonstrated this phenomenon statistically in a group of aphasic patients with intermittent auditory imperception. Patients in this group frequently failed to recognize a common word despite their marked language recovery.

This phenomenon raises a crucial point—that the selection of test materials directly influences the range of responses obtained. The *MTDDA* contains many more items within its subtests than do other diagnostic batteries. This maximizes the opportunity for noticing the on-off effect. This author has used three diagnostic batteries extensively, and interestingly, has only identified patients having this on-off effect using the *MTDDA*.

If a patient's responses are atypical in that he tends to miss easy items and hard items in equal proportion, or he makes errors that are unexpected in terms of the length and complexity of the stimulus offered, the on-off effect should be considered as a possible cause. Administration of a vocabulary test, a spelling test, or any test of at least 20 consecutive items with scaled levels of difficulty, might help identify this phenomenon.

The patient experiences a reduction of information due to slow rise time.[63] Using the *Token Test,* Brookshire[63] identified a group of patients who tended to "miss the initial portion of incoming auditory messages, because the auditory system requires longer than usual to shift from a passive state to an active processing state." [p. 3] He reported that the patient continues to process information efficiently as long as the auditory input continues, but when the input stops and the system returns to a resting state, the first few items will be missed. He added that short commands may be missed in their entirety.

SUMMARY AND CONCLUSIONS

This chapter reviewed certain notions about language and auditory processing, and related this information to the language behavior seen in adult aphasia. The purpose of the review was to illustrate that language processing and auditory processing, while interdependent, do manifest separately, and to point out that some patients with aphasia have, in addition to the language disturbance, an auditory processing disorder.

An auditory processing paradigm was presented to illustrate the intricate relationship between auditory processing and language, and to specify auditory processes that might be identified in the aphasic patient. The idea was developed that an aphasic disorder implies an auditory processing disorder, but that some patients experience a more pervasive and persistent disturbance of the auditory system in addition to that which exists coincident with the aphasia. These patients are not always recognized by scores on language tests and frequently appear to have global aphasia when tested within a few days of the onset of the stroke. A discussion of the various behaviors of these patients on aphasia test batteries illustrated why misclassifications might occur.

Several theoretic notions that illustrate specific auditory processing disorders were discussed and related to the auditory processing paradigm, and to behavior that could be identified during language testing. It was suggested that few of these processes were specific or mutually exclusive, and that a simple and direct relationship to the auditory processing paradigm or to language tests could not be made. It is this author's hope, however, that both the paradigm and the discussions that followed provided a framework for making inferences about possible relationships, and for planning successful therapy techniques.

Not every patient exhibits symptomatology which necessitates such detailed analysis of language behavior. Some brain damage is too extensive for the expectation that a return of functional language will occur with or without therapy. Some brain damage is mild enough that a spontaneous return of language function is likely to occur. Occasionally, patients who have an aphasia of mild to moderate severity will have been spared enough language function to enable them to get along quite well in the environment in which they find themselves. Other patients with aphasia of mild to moderate severity readily respond to traditional therapy methods. It must be stressed, however, that for research purposes, it is essential to measure the primary disturbances of language, and to identify the specific auditory processing disorders that occur. For differential diagnosis of the classifications of aphasia and for planning a program of therapy, it will be necessary for some patients. For these patients, an understanding of both auditory and language processing will make the difference between functional recovery of language and very few language gains.

REFERENCES

1. Macmahon MKC: Modern linguistics and aphasia. Br J Disord Commun 7:54–63, 1972
2. Heilman K: Neuropsychologic changes in the stroke patient. Geriatrics 29:153–160, 1974
3. Goodglass H, Kaplan E: The Assessment of Aphasia and Related Disorders. Philadelphia, Lea & Febiger, 1972, pp61–64
4. Luria AR: Higher Cortical Functions in Man. New York, Basic Books, 1966, p103
5. Hayward RW, Naeser MA, Zatz LM: Cranial computed tomography in aphasia: Correlation of anatomical lesions with functional deficits. Radiology 123:653–660, 1977
6. Karis R, Horenstein S: Localization of speech parameters by brain scans. Neurology 26:226–230, 1976
7. Brain R: Wernicke's Aphasia, in Brain R: Diseases of the Nervous System. New York, Oxford University Press, 1956, p102
8. Critchley M: Head's contribution to aphasia. Brain 84:551–560, 1961
9. Blumstein SE, Baker E, Weintraub S: Phonological factors in auditory comprehension in aphasia. Neuropsychologia 15:19–30, 1977
10. Blumstein S: Some phonological implications of aphasic speech, in Goodglass H, Blumstein S (eds): Psycholinguistics and Aphasia. Baltimore, Johns Hopkins University Press, 1973, pp123–137
11. Goodglass H: Studies on the grammar of aphasics, in Goodglass H, Blumstein S (eds): Psycholinguistics and Aphasia. Baltimore, Johns Hopkins University Press, 1973, pp183–215
12. Goodglass H: Studies on the grammar of aphasics, in Rosenberg S, Koplin JH (eds): Developments in Applied Psycholinguistics Research. New York, Macmillan, 1968, pp177-208
13. Gardner H, Denes G, Zurif E: Critical reading at the sentence level in aphasia. Cortex 11:60–72, 1975
14. Schuell H, Jenkins JH, Jimenez-Pabon E: Aphasia in Adults. New York, Harper & Row, 1964
15. Karasseva TA: The role of the temporal lobe in human auditory perception. Neuropsychologia 10:227–231, 1972
16. Krashen SD: Cerebral asymmetry, in Whitaker H, Whitaker HA (eds): Studies in Neurolinguistics. New York, Academic Press, 1976, pp157–191
17. Blumstein SE: The use and theoretical implications of the dichotic technique for investigating distinctive features. Brain Lang 1:337–350, 1974
18. Johnson RC, Bowers JK, Gamble M, et al: Ability to transcribe music and ear superiority for tone sequences. Cortex 13:295–299, 1977
19. Molfese DL: Neuroelectrical correlates of categorical speech perception in adults. Brain Lang 5:25–35, 1978
20. Tallal P, Newcombe F: Impairment of auditory perception and language comprehension in dysphasia. Brain Lang 5:13–24, 1978
21. Goldberg E, Vaughan H: Nonverbal descriptive systems and hemispheric asymmetry: Shape versus texture discrimination. Brain Lang 5:249–257, 1978
22. Kinsburne M: The minor cerebral hemisphere as a source of aphasic speech. Arch Neurol 25:302–306, 1971
23. Smith A: Speech and other functions after left (dominant) hemispherectomy. J Neurol Neurosurg Psychiatry 29:467–471, 1966
24. Burklund CW: Cerebral hemisphere functions in man: Facts vs. tradition, in Smith WL (ed): Drugs, Development, and Cerebral Function. Springfield, Charles C Thomas, 1972, pp8–36

25. Zaidel E: Auditory vocabulary of the right hemisphere following brain bisection or hemidecortication. Cortex 12:191–211, 1976
26. Zaidel E: Unilateral auditory language comprehension on the token test following cerebral commissurotomy and hemispherectomy. Neuropsychologia 15:1–18, 1977
27. Cullen JK Jr, Thompson CL, Hughes LF, et al: The effects of varied acoustic parameters on performance in dichotic speech perception tasks. Brain Lang 1:307–322, 1974
28. Yorkston KM, Marshall RC, Butler MR: Imposed delay of response: Effects on aphasics' auditory comprehension of visually and nonvisually cued material. Percept Mot Skills 44:647–655, 1977
29. Spreen O: Psycholinguistics and aphasia: The contribution of Arnold Pick, in Goodglass H, Blumstein S (eds): Psycholinguistics and Aphasia. Baltimore, Johns Hopkins University Press, 1973, pp141–170
30. Strub RL, Gardner H: The repetition defect in conduction aphasia: Amnestic or linguistic? Brain Lang 1:241–255, 1974
31. Denes PB, Pinson EN: The Speech Chain. New York, Bell Laboratories, 1969
32. Davis H: Acoustics and psychoacoustics, in Davis H, Silverman S (eds): Hearing and Deafness. New York, Holt, Rinehart and Winston, 1970, pp9–44
33. Carhart R: Development and conservation of speech, in Davis H, Silverman S (eds): Hearing and Deafness. New York, Holt, Rinehart and Winston, 1970, pp360–371
34. Luria AR: Language and brain: Toward the basic problems of neurolinguistics. Brain Lang 1:1–14, 1974
35. Wolf CG: The processing of fundamental frequency in a dichotic matching task. Brain Lang 4:70–77, 1977
36. Ojemann GA: Organization of short-term verbal memory in language areas of human cortex: Evidence from electrical stimulation. Brain Lang 5:331–340, 1978
37. Luria AR: The Working Brain. New York, Basic Books, 1973, p137
38. Shallice T, Warrington EK: The dissociation between short-term retention of meaningful sounds and verbal material. Neuropsychologia 12:553–555, 1974
39. Locke JL, Deck JW: Retrieval failure, rehearsal deficiency and short-term memory loss in the aphasic adult. Brain Lang 5:227–235, 1978
40. Kintsch W: Learning, Memory, and Conceptual Processes. New York, John Wiley & Sons, 1970, pp157–162
41. Cermak LS, Moreines J: Verbal retention deficits in aphasic and amnestic patients. Brain Lang 3:16–27, 1976
42. Coughlan AK, Warrington EK: Word comprehension and word retrieval in patients with localized cerebral lesions. Brain 101:163–185, 1978
43. Laver J: Language and nonverbal communication, in Carterette EC, Friedman MP (eds): Handbook of Perception, vol VII. (Language and Speech) New York, Academic Press, 1976, pp345–361
44. Howes D: Some experimental investigations of language in aphasia, in Salzinger S (ed): Research in Verbal Behavior and Some Neurophysiological Implications. New York, Academic Press, 1967, pp181–199
45. Schuell H, Johnston KL: Unpublished data, 1970
46. Schuell H: Minnesota Test for Differential Diagnosis of Aphasia (rev ed). Minneapolis, University of Minnesota Press, 1972
47. Porch BE: Porch Index of Communicative Ability (rev ed). Palo Alto, Consulting Psychologists Press, 1971
48. Spreen O, Benton AL: Neurosensory Center Comprehensive Examination for Aphasia (rev ed). Victoria, British Columbia, University of Victoria, 1969
49. Schuell H: Intermittent Auditory Imperception. (Lecture, 1966)

50. De Renzi E, Vignolo LA: The Token Test: A sensitive test to detect receptive disturbances in aphasics. Brain 85:665–678, 1962
51. Crockett DJ: Multivariate comparison of Howes' and Weisenburg and McBride's models of aphasia on the Neurosensory Center Comprehensive Examination. Percept Mot Skills 43: 795–806, 1976
52. Harris CM: Phonemic Errors Made by Aphasic Subjects in the Identification of Monosyllabic Words. Ph.D. Thesis, University of Minnesota, 1970, Unpublished
53. Geschwind N: Correct concepts: Aphasia. N Engl J Med 284:654–656, 1971
54. Buckingham HW, Jr, Kertesz A: A linguistic study of fluent aphasia. Brain Lang 1:43–62, 1974
55. Beyn ES, Vlasenko IT: Verbal paraphasias of aphasic patients in the course of naming actions. Br J Disord Commun 9:24–34, 1974
56. Goodglass H, Klein B, Carey P, Jones KJ: Specific semantic word categories in aphasia, in Goodglass H, Blumstein S (eds): Psycholinguistics and Aphasia. Baltimore, Johns Hopkins University Press, 1973, pp250–266
57. Brown JW: The problem of repetition: A study of "conduction" aphasia and the "isolation" syndrome. Cortex 11:37–52, 1975
58. Olson GM, Clark HH: Research methods in psycholinguistics, in Carterette ED, Friedman MP (eds): Handbook of Perception, vol VII. (Language and Speech) New York, Academic Press, 1976, pp25–74
59. Gardner H, Albert ML, Weintraub S: Comprehending a word: The influence of speed and redundancy on auditory comprehension in aphasia. Cortex 11:155–162, 1975
60. Rudnick KJ, Berry RC: Perception of rate-altered sentential approximations by normal and aphasic children. Percept Mot Skills 40:703–709, 1975
61. Natale M: Perception of nonlinguistic auditory rhythms by the speech hemisphere. Brain Lang 4:32–44, 1977
62. Hirsh IJ: Auditory training, in Davis H, Silverman S (eds): Hearing and Deafness. New York, Holt, Rinehart and Winston, 1970, pp346–359
63. Brookshire R: Differences in responding to auditory verbal materials among aphasic patients. Acta Symbol 5:1–18, 1974
64. Schuell H: Personal notes, 1965

Kathleen L. Johnston

9

Auditory Processing Disorders and Aphasic Adults: Diagnosis and Treatment

In order to identify impaired cerebral processes which result in language disorders, information must be gathered. The observation of behavior, the administration of informal and standardized tests, and the review of case histories are done for the purpose of arriving at a diagnosis that will suggest the next course of action for patient and therapist. Sometimes this information can be obtained leisurely: the patient feels well and tolerates a battery of tests that can be administered over a period of days or weeks. Frequently, however, diagnosis is necessary while the patient is still in the hospital and before he begins to feel fit.

THE ACUTELY ILL PATIENT

Differentiating the types of aphasia in acutely ill patients is difficult at best, and, when the patient has severe involvement of auditory processes in addition to language disturbance, it sometimes appears impossible. Acutely ill patients often do not score normally on language tests whether language disorders exist or not.[1] Low test scores may reflect the fact that the brain as a whole is not working normally; this does not necessarily mean that language is impaired. Ordinarily, acutely ill patients are unable to attend to test materials for longer than a few minutes, and this lack of attention is reflected in test scores. Confused patients sometimes exhibit disturbances of memory and thought that affect their performances on language tests. A distraught patient may begin a test, but as item difficulty increases, the patient's tension rises and he may refuse to finish the task. Patients with visual disorders have problems seeing the test materials. Patients with one paralyzed arm and one arm attached to an intravenous feeding apparatus cannot write, and have trouble pointing to materials. Even elderly normal subjects may make errors on language tests.[1] Many of these subjects digress into other areas, perseverate, and confuse test directions. Like acutely ill patients, they tend to reject reading and writing tasks by complaining of poor vision, arthritis, and exhaustion. Therefore, when acutely ill patients are tested, it is important to remember that it is not the *number* of errors, but the *patterns* and *types* of errors that are diagnostically important.

The number of days post onset after which the test is administered is of critical importance when conclusions about classification of aphasia are made. Generally, patients who are tested within seven days post onset are considered acutely ill. Patients tested from 10 to 15 days post onset can be considered neurophysiologically stable. Patients tested from three to six months post onset are usually considered stable. Classifications as to type of aphasia are not reliable when made before three months post onset, but some initial diagnoses are less reliable than others. In a study designed by Schuell, it was found that acutely ill patients who tended to be misclassified most frequently were those with involvement of multiple processes, with global aphasia, or with severe auditory processing disorders.[1]

When a patient performs minimally or not at all on a test battery, it may be an indication of critical illess. In a study done by Rubens, Ramirez-Lassepas, and Johnston,[2] 48.5 percent of patients who could not be tested because they responded only minimally to the testing situation (in spite of being awake and alert) died within three months of the stroke without recovering any functional speech. These patients were suffering bilateral hemispherical infarctions or massive unilateral involvement, and their mortality was much higher than that for all cerebral infarctions.

Critically ill patients should not be badgered with complex language batteries. Severely involved, less ill patients should be reassured that help with speech and language will be available to them when they are feeling better. When an acutely ill patient is seen, guidance from the medical staff notes as to the patient's physical status should be a primary consideration in determining just how much formalized testing should be accomplished during the initial visit. Very often the critically ill patient will smile and acknowledge the examiner, and attend to the test materials presented to him. But usually, he cannot be enticed to perform on test items. His behavior seems to say, "I don't wish to be rude and I know you are trying to help, but I can't be bothered with this just now."

Observation of behavior is extremely important when attempting to separate the effects of the illness from the language disturbance. For example, patients with global aphasia, if they are alert and not too ill, will often show evidence of interest in the examiner and in the test. They attempt to cooperate, they try to perform tasks when encouraged, and they may respond correctly to easier test items. Often they seem to recognize that their responses are incorrect. Their behavior suggests that they are trying their best, but that they find the material too difficult for them to perform as expected.

Another kind of acutely ill patient, who offers minimal or no response to a test battery, is the one with severe auditory disorder, jargon, euphoria, and copious verbal output. This patient rarely attends to the speaker, but seems to be earnestly trying to explain something about himself. He resists most attempts to focus his attention on a task, and places himself in the center of attention. Rochford[3] presents an excellent description of this patient and provides good evidence that the aphasia is part of a wider syndrome which includes disturbances of insight, mood, and orientation. Rochford believes that the mood disturbances are primary and probably reflect injury to the nondominant hemisphere. The patients he describes have anosognosia—a lack of awareness of their deficit and of insight into their problem. They also have euphoria and exhibit social disinhibition. They may respond to test items by saying, "I know what that is, so why am I taking this silly test?" One such patient refused to repeat or to read the phrase, 'white snow'. He explained, "It says, it is, well, you know I know what it is. It is outside. Cold." He added gestures to his description to prove his point. He could not be made to understand that his inability to express the phrase, either by reading it or repeating it after the examiner, indicated a language problem. Such remarks during testing and therapy should be documented because they are often clues to the presence of this syndrome. These patients do not respond well to therapy because the anosognosia remains even after they become stable.

Sometimes patients with severe auditory processing disorders do not respond to testing because they do not realize that they have a problem understanding others, or a problem saying words so that others can understand them. One patient who had been extremely uncooperative later explained that she would never have been so mean to everyone if just one person had explained to her why she was in the hospital. She explained: "I felt fine, and as far as I could see, there was nothing the matter with me." Initially, this patient had severe aphasia and a severe auditory processing disorder; she could not tell that her own speech was unintelligible, and she could not understand the explanations offered by her doctors and family. Some of these patients may believe that there is nothing wrong with their speech, and that hospital personnel are simply refusing to understand them. Other patients seem to believe that if there is anything wrong with their speech, it is minor. They believe that if the listener just thought about it a little, they could be understood. Initially, these feelings are exhibited in hostility of varying degrees. This hostile behavior may be a clue that a severe auditory processing disorder is present.

The list of different types of patients who respond minimally or not at all to language tests is neither definitive nor exhaustive. It is presented here to stress the point that acutely ill patients do not always respond to language tests. Unless some arrangement for follow-up is made at the time of initial testing, these patients may be lost to language pathologists when they are discharged to facilities that do not offer rehabilitative services. If, as it seems, there are identifiable patterns of behavior that reflect prognosis and classification in these patients, we must begin to differentiate them. Most patients with auditory processing disorders can improve with therapy, and most facilities will cooperate in rehabilitative efforts instigated by the referring hospital. There may be valid reasons for not offering therapy to a particular patient, but a patient should not be denied therapy because of misclassification resulting from minimal test responses obtained before he was stable.

DIFFERENTIAL DIAGNOSIS

The procedures and techniques necessary and available for differential diagnosis have not yet evolved into a science. Conclusions about the classification of aphasia in a particular patient might vary according to the severity of aphasia,[4] the number of days post onset, the time of day the test was administered, the test batteries selected,[5] and examiner or test author bias.[4, 5] The examiner's approach to the testing situation is influenced by individual differences among patients in both symptomatology and personality. Examiners draw upon a variety of experiences in attempting to elicit responses. What works with one examiner may not be very effective in a similar instance with another. Therefore, the ideas about diagnosis and therapy outlined in this chapter are guidelines to be followed, modified, or dismissed entirely, as warranted by the situation.

Observe Behavior

The first step in differential diagnosis is to note behavior. The development of behavioral scales may eventually be incorporated into aphasia testing procedures, but until that time, those who work with acutely ill and/or severely involved patients must follow their own guidelines for noting behavior. The preliminary results of one study[2] suggest that one can predict the outcome for certain groups of patients from their general testing behavior. Patients who respond neither to the examiner nor to the test, or to the examiner but not to the test, or to both the examiner and the test without maintaining test performance, are usually acutely or critically ill. They have limited chances for recovery of language function. Their chances for recovery, however, do increase as sustained interest in the test items increases. Patients who are responsive and cooperative but who make few or no correct responses to the test items, have an even chance of regaining some language. Patients who are responsive and cooperative to parts of the test but refuse many test items, or patients who perform the test battery, will recover a degree of language commensurate with the kind of aphasia that exists. Ideally, even the first group of patients mentioned, those who are acutely ill, should be followed at monthly intervals for the first three months, and again at six months post onset, for observation of any behavioral changes that may warrant further evaluation. Patients in the third group, those who perform the test battery, have test scores which are prognostic and usually provide sufficient basis for therapy plans. Patients in the second group, those who are responsive and cooperative but make few correct responses, present the majority of diagnostic problems.

Analyze Incorrect Responses

This situation relates to the second step in differential diagnosis, to analyze incorrect responses. There are many diagnostic gradations among incorrect responses on test items. Most test batteries allow for either minimal or no analysis of incorrect answers. While the right or wrong scoring technique makes scoring much simpler, it is not diagnostic. The most pertinent information for differential diagnosis often is gleaned from what the patient says and does while attempting to respond. The *Minnesota Test for Differential Diagnosis of Aphasia* (MTDDA)[6] allows for annotation of semantic, auditory, visual, or random associations on two of its subtests. The *Boston Diagnostic Aphasia Examination* (BDAE)[7] allows the examiner to mark and count various paraphasias that occur, and to score on the basis of processing time on several of its subtests. The *Neurosensory Center Comprehensive Examination for Aphasia* (NCCEA)[8] takes note of error types on naming tasks. The *Porch Index of Communicative Ability* (PICA)[9] offers a scoring system delineating gradations of responses, and is the only one of these mentioned to have a consistent and systematic method of analyzing incorrect responses as to severity and type.*

*Discussions of additional tests of general language ability can be found in articles by Eisenson[25] and Wertz.[56]

Usually, a sophisticated analysis is not necessary because aphasia classification systems are concerned with relationships between the skills a patient does and does not possess. Simply noting the patterns of strengths and weaknesses, the inconsistencies of responses, and the comparisons across modalities of language (listening, speaking, reading, and writing), offers sufficient information for a tentative, but workable diagnosis.

In addition to noting processing time, paraphasic errors, and association errors, other behaviors should be noted in the test booklets. Does the patient have more difficulty with one part of speech than with another? Does he ask for repetitions of the directions or the stimuli? Is spontaneous speech superior to speech during test performance? Writing down all responses, even when incorrect, offers clues as to the patient's processing behavior. A patient who answers "eleven" when asked how many things are in a dozen may understand the question and arrive at his answer by counting up to twelve and stopping one number too soon. A patient who answers, "It depends on what you want," probably did not understand the question. Writing down patient responses need not interfere with either testing procedures or rapport. With practice, it can be done quickly and unobtrusively. Sometimes a patient appears to be responding randomly, but his responses form a pattern when these behaviors are collected and reviewed.

Inquiries as to whether the patient is comfortable or has difficulty seeing or hearing, often elicit elaborate, helpful gestures. One patient who appeared to be pointing to the first item that came to his attention with the seeming aim of finishing the test as rapidly as possible, was asked, "Are you comfortable?" The patient blushed and said no and pointed to the bathroom. It was the only word elicited during the entire test, but once he had used the bathroom, his responses became significantly more consistent.

Look for Patterns

A third step in differential diagnosis is to examine the items refused for a pattern. Patients refuse items for a variety of reasons, ranging from discomfort to item difficulty. Encourage the patient to attempt an explanation for his refusal. Patients are generally able to indicate that they are tired, worried, or uncomfortable. Some patients tend to stop performing as test difficulty increases. Other patients may describe an ailment or disease that prevents their performance on specific tests. The examiner who has the courage to ask polite but pointed questions, and the patience to try and understand the answers, can be rewarded with diagnostic information. For example, one patient who refused many test items, when given the opportunity, explained his test performance by describing by word and gesture an unusual variety of hemianopia (visual field defect) which had been missed on the initial neurologic evaluation.

Improvise to Obtain a Response

A fourth step in differential diagnosis is to improvise until a response is obtained. Patients who don't respond well to tests still enjoy visitors; they enjoy showing off pictures of children, cards from friends, or a treasured possession. A conversation can be built around any of these things, and inferences can be made as to comprehension, vocabulary level, and expressive ability.

For purposes of research, it is very important for examiners to adhere rigidly to test directions. But once the subtest has been administered and scored, it is sometimes necessary to return to the item and administer it in any way possible to elicit a response. For example, if a patient has a severe auditory processing disorder and does not respond to any of the auditory tests, he offers no clue as to the specific type of processing problem he may have. The clinician might cover all but two or three pictured objects and tell the patient that he should point to the one named. If the patient is not sure about his answer, he should be encouraged to guess. This technique of returning to a subtest and experimenting until a response is obtained can be very revealing for the examiner. One patient, who had not understood the test directions and who did not wish to appear foolish, smiled delightedly, said, "Oh," and responded correctly to the remainder of the subtest items. It is important to remember that a, 'no response', cannot be analyzed. First, the test must be administered properly and then, partially readministered with the idea of obtaining a response.

Some aphasia test batteries are quite lenient when it comes to offering the patient feedback as to whether he is making errors. These batteries allow the examiner to give cues to the patient so that he can achieve some success. Patients perform much better when they have some feedback about whether they are performing as expected. Tests which allow this feedback are preferred if analysis of behavior is required for a differential diagnosis.

The regulated format of some tests is too rigid for some patients; they become discouraged with their failures and stop performing. A patient can be taught to respond to some of the easier test items, although the responses can not be scored. This relieves his frustration with the test and offers the examiner more samples of behavior on which to base his conclusions. Also, this approach makes the patient more willing to attempt the test again at a later date.

Administer Additional Tests

Sometimes for diagnosis and for construction of a program of therapy, a fifth step is necessary, to administer additional tests. Examples of tests that are useful in identifying auditory processing disorders include the following:

1. Picture vocabulary tests such as the Ammon's[10] or Peabody.[11] Unlike other types of aphasic patients, those with auditory processing disorders tend to miss easier items and respond correctly to more difficult items.
2. Spelling tests like those from the *Wide Range Achievement Test*.[12] The large number of times gives the examiner an opportunity to note the on-off effect. (See Chapter 7). Patients with auditory processing disorders tend to perform inconsistently. For example, a patient who misses words like 'he,' 'her,' 'and,' and 'but,' but accurately spells longer, more difficult words, may well be unable to perceive the shorter words. In addition, patients may make auditory errors, correctly writing a different word that sounds like the one given.
3. Reading tests such as the *Gates-MacGinitie Reading Tests*.[13] Some patients with auditory processing disorders exhibit more comprehension on reading tasks in comparison to similar auditory tasks. Patients with more severe auditory processing disorders may make linguistic errors on reading tests that are similar to the errors they make on auditory tests.
4. Tests of auditory discrimination such as the *Wepman Test* of *Auditory Discrimination*.[14]
5. The *Token Test*.[15] This test was designed to detect subtle disorders in the ability to understand spoken language.
6. Examples of other tests for auditory functioning can be found in the *Detroit Tests of Learning Aptitude*[16] or the *Illinois Test of Psycholinguistic Abilities*.[17]

There is no magic formula for analyzing and integrating test results into a definitive diagnosis, but scores and behavioral observations should reveal areas of deficit which, in turn, suggest therapy techniques. A diagnosis will evolve over time. More important than a diagnostic word is an accurate and complete description of behavior.

Initiate Diagnostic Therapy

A sixth step which may become necessary with severely involved patients is to initiate a period of diagnostic therapy. During his time a compromise is made between the patient's need to understand this problem and begin a program of rehabilitation, and the therapist's need to experiment with procedures based on the results of a variety of additional tests. Diagnostic therapy might extend from two days to two weeks or more. Actually all therapy is diagnostic in that it continually reveals areas of performance that were unpredicted. After two weeks some definitive therapy plan should be stated and initiated. For patients who are difficult to diagnose, it becomes extremely important to keep a record of all responses (Fig. 9-1). Every therapy tech-

Stimulus: Sentence, phrase, word, object, syllable or phoneme

	MON.	TUES.	WED.	THURS.	FRI.
1.					
2.					
3.					
4.					
5.					
6.					
7.					
8.					
9.					
10.					
11.					
12.					
13.					
14.					
15.					
16.					
17.					
18.					
19.					
20.					

Task presented: repetition
discrimination
recognition
verbalization
reading
copying (stimulus presented, then removed)
writing to dictation
other:

Fig. 9-1. A chart that can be used for keeping a record of the responses made during diagnostic therapy.

nique should be specified and used until it can be discarded with an explanation as to why it was or was not successful. This documentation can prevent the waste of hours of therapy time spent using techniques and procedures inappropriate to the specific aphasic problem.

Complicating Conditions

Another factor influencing differential diagnosis is the presence of conditions complicating the aphasia. For example, a patient who is deaf may not be able to hear the test directions or stimuli; a blind patient cannot read. Many stroke victims have difficulty with vision due to visual field defects or to visual acuity problems. These patients have difficulty reading and writing. Errors related to visual processing disorders exist and can be separated from auditory processing errors. Patients may also have problems with memory, orientation, and insight, or they may present psychotic-like behavior.

Another complicating factor that can be present is apraxia—the inability to immediately assume the correct positions of tongue and lips, which results in substitutions for individual articulations. There is no paralysis of the oral speech musculature. The tongue behaves as though it doesn't know where to go because of a disturbance of kinesthetic movement.[18]* Oral apraxia is a confusing phenomena because it usually does not exist in isolation. It is called by various names,[20] and it can be difficult to distinguish from motor aphasia. This is not surprising because the two often occur together. Some authors have suggested that apractic difficulties are due to a reduction of auditory and proprioceptive information.[21] Others state that apractic errors do not have their basis in auditory perceptual impairment.[22] Perhaps an appropriate summary of the situation is offered by Macmahon[23] who states that the relationship between phonetic disintegration and apraxia is not yet fully understood.

Apraxia can exist in conjunction with aphasia and auditory processing disorders. Sometimes patients with auditory processing disorders are mistakenly classified as having apraxia because the phonetic integration of their speech is severely disrupted. This classification confusion tends to occur primarily when patients have multiple, severe processing disorders, and when they are unable to respond definitively to tests of oral apraxia which are incorporated into the language test battery.[24] To minimize this confusion, a general examination for apraxia that includes some evaluation of the oral speech musculature should be done. Examples of tests for apraxia include requesting the patient to show how to use a toothbrush, how to light a cigarette, or how to blow out a match. Personal experience suggests that patients with multiple

*For a thorough delineation of the dysarthrias and apraxia, see Darley *et al.*[19]

involvements respond well to long-term therapy if the factors contributing to their speech and language problems are isolated and treated accordingly (usually separately).

TRADITIONAL THERAPY TECHNIQUES

The efficacy of language rehabilitation for adult aphasic patients is a vital professional issue. The literature includes accounts which suggest that therapy does enhance language recovery.[25-27] But until a practical method is found to separate the effects of therapy from those of spontaneous recovery,[28-30] there is no objective rationale for who should or should not receive therapy, for when they should receive it, and for how long it should be offered.[31] Most aphasiologists believe that patients who have not suffered extensive and irreversible brain damage can benefit from therapy. Some believe that it is not the effect of specific treatment procedures that yields improvement, but the more general integrational effect of the course of treatment.[32]

There is no universally agreed upon system for speech and language stimulation. Therapy techniques are as individual as patients who exhibit language problems. Traditional therapy consists of exercises designed to stimulate language through the use of intensive, repetitive, and controlled auditory stimulation and the feedback processes from obtained responses. For each patient this stimulation begins at the level where the language breakdown occurs, and proceeds systematically from easy to more difficult levels.

Picture-word Card Approach

The majority of patients who can phonate but who have little or no functional speech respond to the traditional picture-word card approach. The Language Master[33] and the sets of cards designed for building vocabulary may be used, or therapists may design their own materials. With this technique, from 10 to 20 cards of a series are chosen for each week's work. The patient hears the word, responds by pointing to the correct picture, and attempts to repeat the word. Usually the patient begins to repeat after the first few exposures to the cards, and his responses become closer approximations to the target word as stimulations increase. The patient is also requested to first copy the word, then write it to dictation, and ultimately write it upon presentation of the picture. He is encouraged to use the word in phrases and short sentences. Therapy proceeds by replacing the pictures with words, and the words with short sentences.

For increasing his retention span, the patient might point to objects, pictures or words in series of two, three or more. As retention span increases, patients are asked to respond to complex commands. As spontaneous speech develops, patients might answer simple questions, use words in sentences, define words, and describe the events in selected action pictures. Words, objects, and pictures are not chosen randomly but according to guidelines. For example, words may be chosen because of their frequency of use in the language, because they are geared to the patient's particular environment, or because they contain sounds that are easier for the patient to produce. Whatever the choice, the same words are used repeatedly until the patient responds to them easily, after which new words are chosen.

Multisensory Techniques

Severely or multiply involved patients often benefit from multisensory techniques—the coordination of hand, eye, and ear with movements of the speech musculature. For example, as the hand holds the figure of a chair, the eye can observe it and the printed word, and the ear can hear the word repeated, sometimes as many as 20 times. Tracing shapes, numbers, letters, and words while saying or listening to their names, often is successful initially in eliciting responses. For some severely involved patients, Melodic Intonation Therapy[34] is a good example of a successful multisensory approach.

Ideally, therapy continues until the patient has enough language to communicate effectively in his environment. Most rehabilitatable patients admitted to therapy achieve this point between six and nine months after the onset of the stroke. Although additional therapy can contribute further gains in language function, these gains are often minimal and frequently do not warrant the cost and commitment necessary to continue therapy. Occasionally, patients with extraordinary drive and determination attain a high level of improvement with long-term therapy, and may even be able to return to jobs held before the stroke.

A THERAPY PROGRAM FOR PATIENTS WITH AUDITORY PROCESSING DISORDERS

There are patients with auditory processing disorders who respond well to the traditional therapy described above. Patients with severe auditory processing disturbances, however, tend to react poorly to these techniques. They appear puzzled by the bombardment of auditory stimulation. Even the most elementary speech units seem confusing unless they are presented in a highly structured manner. For these patients, materials must be presented in such a way that auditory input is drastically reduced, rigidly controlled, and accompanied by a variety of nonauditory cues. Such limitation of auditory input allows the patient the opportunity to focus on a specific target within a range of possibilities. Limiting and structuring input reduces the number of percepts to which the patient must listen,[35] and reduces the possibility of overloading the auditory system.

Patients with auditory receptive difficulties also appear to have a deficit in categorizing auditory stimuli.[35, 36] Therapy for these patients should provide methods to assist the categorization process, visual and tactile cues to accompany the verbal presentation, and limited auditory input. The linguistic chart technique (LCT) was developed to meet these criteria. It has been useful with aphasic patients of any type whose symptomatology is severe, but it is particularly useful with patients who have auditory processing disorders.

The linguistic chart is not one, but many charts, each devised according to the patient's linguistic needs. It begins on the level of single sounds with application of distinctive feature analysis as the linguistic principle, and proceeds to syllables and words of increasing complexity. Charts of more complex functioning, such as those based on the morphologic or syntactic structure of the language, can also be constructed. The framework provided by linguistic principles allows the therapist to select and diagram specified items for presentation and to build upon the items in a highly structured manner. The use of colored symbols, figures, and diacritical marks may be added for visual cueing of the auditory input. Initially, this technique can be used in conjunction with the more traditional therapy approach. But as the patient finds the LCT less frustrating and more rewarding, more therapy time should be devoted to it.

The LCT came into existence primarily through trial and error, and has been modified as more knowledge of linguistics and its application to language disorders has accumulated. Its evolution is not complete; there has been little experimentation with controlling the lexicon with regard to parts of speech presented,[37-39] and the underlying theory regarding distinctive features needs refinement.[40] But despite these limitations, the LCT has been successful because of the combined effects of reducing and controlling inputs, of providing a variety of nonauditory cues, of organizing a well-ordered linguistic progression, and of proceeding at a pace suited to individual needs.

THE LINGUISTIC CHART TECHNIQUE

Patient Selection

The patients for whom the LCT was designed are patients who have language and auditory processing dysfunction as a result of a lesion which includes the temporal cortex of the left (dominant) hemisphere. Language and supplementary tests indicate the presence of defective recognition of the sounds of speech. Frequently, the patient is unable to correctly respond at the single word level. These patients usually present severe symptomatology, may have oral apraxia, and usually do not regain speech without therapy.[37, 41]

Therapy Goals

The purpose of the LCT is to assist the patient in his analysis of the sound composition of words. This is accomplished by separating the individual sounds within words using the auditory modality, and then recombining the sounds into word groups to assist the classification process through visual cueing.[37, 41]

Eliciting Speech Sounds

LCT therapy begins with the elicitation of a sound. Patients who are unable to reproduce a recognizable speech sound at will may need to proceed from a sigh, cough, or grunt. Often the first sounds produced by the patient are distorted when compared to sounds of speech. Accept the sound produced and have the patient experiment with it until it more closely approximates the desired sound. You might draw a diagram of the position of the tongue in the mouth when the sound is produced, or diagrams representing alterations made by changing the position of the oral speech musculature. Illustrations of the oral speech musculature found in a variety of texts may be very useful. There are other techniques which may be used. Mirrors offer the patient feedback as to how his lips and tongue are positioned; manipulation of the tongue with a tongue depressor offers the patient tactile feedback about the correct tongue position. A diagram usually is a sufficient cue for most patients. What is important to remember is that the patient initially needs a visual cue in order to consistently produce a correct response.

When a reasonable approximation of a speech sound is elicited, repeat the entire elicitation process as many times as necessary for the patient to begin to reproduce the sound. When the patient is able to repeat the sound and produce it spontaneously, label the diagram with a name for the sound. There are alphabets modified to assure a correspondence between sound and symbol that have been used successfully with learning disabled children.[42] It is acceptable to use these with aphasic patients. The phonetic alphabet, however, works very well; usually it is not distracting to the patients, and it represents sounds practiced in therapy. It ultimately becomes a visual cue for the patient's response (Fig. 9-2). Some kind of notation system must be used because the patient is not able to discriminate the differences between the sounds an individual letter makes. Without a visual cue, the entire therapy process may take considerably longer than necessary.

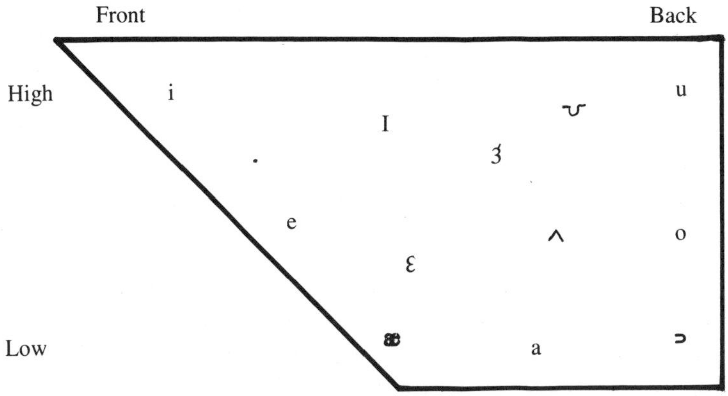

i	meet	ɝ	churn	u	fool
I	mit	ʌ	judge	ʊ	full
e	mate	a	father	o	foal
ɛ	met			ɔ	fall
æ	mat				

Fig. 9-2. Chart of English Vowel Phonemes

Add sounds using a diagram to point out lip rounding and tongue position, and accept the next different sound that the patient can consistently produce. Diagram the position of the new sound and label it. Then have the patient produce each sound repeatedly, each time associating the appropriate diagram to the corresponding sound. Continue practicing with the patient producing the sounds and identifying them by diagram, and the therapist producing the sounds and having the patient identify them by diagram.

After several practice sessions the patient should no longer need to refer to the diagram. The diagram can then be replaced by the letter representing the sound. Letters representing vowels typify more than one sound. Therefore, the letter should be accompanied by the phonetic symbol written as a subscript or in parentheses. Since patients usually acquire /æ/ as in 'hat', or /a/ as in 'father', before /e/ as in 'plane',* the diacritical marks for long and short vowels are not sufficient to differentiate the various sounds one letter may make. Usually, only two to four sounds need to be worked on in this manner. After the initial few days of practice on the first two or three, the patient is able to produce and identify many others, more quickly and easily.

*The order of acquisition is similar to that found in patients classified as having Broca's aphasia, with the low vowels easier to acquire than the high vowels.[43]

VOWELS

Often, it is a vowel sound that patients find easiest to produce initially. There is evidence in the literature suggesting that the acoustic features that act as cues for perception differ for vowels and certain consonants, and that the feature which seems to be of the greatest assistance to aphasic patients is the front-back contrast (Fig. 9-2).[44] There is evidence that vowels, nasals, and liquids (see Table 8-3, p 149 for a graphic description of terms) require less acoustic restructuring, and therefore, may be less dependent upon specialized left hemisphere mechanisms for analysis.[45] In addition, Trost and Canter[46] report that patients with apraxia make fewer errors on vowel production than on single consonants. Their data was gathered on patients having Broca's aphasia, and it is possible that it would not be replicated with the patients under discussion.

Patients who find vowels easier to produce initially may experience some difficulty incorporating all of the vowel sounds into their spontaneous production. They may find /e/, /i/, and /ai/ very difficult to produce early in therapy because they do not seem to hear the transitions involved in producing these sounds, and visual cueing is not precise enough to offer the necessary assistance. If this is the case, work on consonants before all vowel sounds are elicited. Patients usually will begin to use them correctly without further work of the nature described above.

CONSONANTS

There is evidence in the literature that consonants, particularly stop consonants, require relatively more left hemisphere processing than vowels.[45, 47] The patients for whom the LCT was designed have considerable difficulty differentiating among the stop consonants, and progress more quickly in therapy when the production of the consonant is stressed, rather than the perceptual recognition. The visual and/or tactile cues presented, together with the feedback received from production attempts, make these sounds easier to mimic than sounds that cannot be seen so easily. It is possible that this regulated practice in production formulates a program for behavior enabling the patient to move from an automatic mode of response (which is now nonfunctional) into a learned function. The patient establishes a hierarchical structure of choices not based upon his auditory perception, but based on development of a cognitive process[48] which allows him to more accurately identify the phoneme which he does not adequately perceive. Initially, it seems that the patient learns substitute skills (for example, in the discrimination of /k/ from /t/) to replace or assist the impaired auditory perceptual skills. He may be incorporating the motor response of saying the sound with the visual representation of the sound in a manner which allows him more awareness of the relationships among sounds, similar to the relationships outlined in a linguistic chart. Auditory discrimination of related sounds improves as the patient develops more refined guessing techniques, and his auditory perceptual responses contain fewer errors as a result of this process.

Therapy methods for consonants are the same as for vowels. Begin with a sound that the patient can produce consistently. This is usually /m/ although some patients have difficulty with the feature of nasality. Some patients find it easier to work with a family of sounds like the bilabials /p/, /b/, and /m/, while others respond better when the second sound to be acquired is one quite different from the first (e.g., /p/ to /k/, or /p/ to /s/).

Diagrams of the positions of the oral speech musculature are usually unnecessary for consonants. Demonstration by the therapist is sufficient to elicit the voiceless bilabial, the labiodental and the interdental sounds. Diacritical marks also are usually unnecessary, although if a patient continues to have difficulty with the variations of the production of a sound (/l/ for example), they may be used. Usually patients quickly acquire enough sounds to allow them to begin to work on syllables and words. The sounds that are difficult will come more easily later in therapy.

SYLLABLES

After four to five sounds have been acquired they may be placed into syllables, and work on production and auditory discrimination of groups of sounds may begin. Syllables can be written on cards, one syllable to a card, and new cards added gradually, one or two at a time. Initially, the patient only needs to point to syllables spoken by the therapist. To do this, mark letters representing the known consonants and vowels on index cards and present them to the patient as shown in Figure 9-3. At this point the procedure is the same as that used in traditional therapy; the patient listens to the syllable (word, phrase, sentence) while he looks at the written representation, and then selects the correct response. In addition to pointing, he should imitate the response (saying the stimulus with the examiner), repeat the response, and write it.

B	E	P	E	M	E
B	A	P	A	M	A
D	E	T	E	N	E

Fig. 9-3.

be	day
we	gay
he	hay
me	jay
she	Kay
key	lay
	may
	pay
	ray
	say

Fig. 9-4.

As the patient improves, sounds may be added as shown in Figure 9-4. As the patient masters more sounds and the cards become time consuming to handle, they can be replaced by a sheet of paper with the vowels written horizontally across the page, and the consonants written vertically. If the patient finds consonants easier to produce, proceed down the page using the vowel sound that comes easiest for him, for example, ba, da, fa, ga, ha. Then proceed across the page, selecting one consonant, until the patient is able to produce it with most vowel sounds, for example, ba, be, bi, bo, bu. Any sound can be omitted or added as the patient is better able to handle it. If the patient is unable to produce a particular sound, accept the response offered, but label it so that he is aware that an adjustment needs to be made to produce the correct response. It is important that the patient receives continuous feedback about his performance.

It is seldom necessary to spend more than 10 to 20 minutes a session for a period of one to three weeks on the entire process of vowels, consonants, and syllables. Most patients begin to handle the auditory stimuli within days of the initiation of this approach. Patients with apraxia in addition to an auditory processing disorder, require more time on sounds and syllables (as outlined in Figures 9-4 and 9-5), but this work can be accomplished in conjunction with

bead	beak	deal	bleed	squeal
knead	leak	heal	breed	steal
lead	peak	meal	creed	clean
mead	teak	peal	greed	glean
read		seal		scream
		real		
		zeal		

Fig. 9-5.

the use of words made up of sounds the patient is able to produce. The patient with apraxia needs more rigid control exerted over the sounds chosen for practice, as well as more practice with sequencing the sounds.[49] Charts such as the ones represented in Figure 9-2 and Table 8-3 enable the therapist to be aware at all times of sounds with maximal and minimal contrasts.

Other patients who may need more practice and more control exerted over the choice of sounds used might be those with severe auditory processing disorders or those with multiple involvements. These patients benefit from practice on word lists like those in Figures 9-4 and 9-5. The lists may be read vertically or horizontally, and new sounds may be added to the words used. All possible vowel and consonant combinations are not necessarily used with each patient. After a period of practice on certain difficult sound combinations, patients begin to find other combinations easier to produce and recognize. It is advantageous to have word charts on hand, however, because individual patients differ with regard to the ease with which they can produce different sounds. A word list that works well for one patient may be very difficult for another.

WORDS

Many patients are able to benefit from the more traditional therapy methods after working on sounds and syllables. They move directly to phrases, sentences, and spontaneous speech. Others may need more practice and benefit from work on word lists (Fig. 9-5 and 9-6). Some patients seem to benefit from the incorporation of known sounds into two syllable words in order to practice making speedy transitions of the oral speech musculature (Fig. 9-6). Neither the spelling nor the meaning of the word is important at this time. This training is used only for practice on movement and sound patterns. It is not necessarily a therapy technique for aphasia, and it is used only five or ten minutes of the therapy sessions.

between	compact	forgive
canteen	contact	outlive
fourteen	impact	outbid
routine	detract	undid
marine		
sardine		

Fig. 9-6.

Discriminating, Reading and Writing Words, Phrases and Sentences

The LCT assists the patient in his ability to recognize, discriminate, and produce sounds. It allows him to perceive visually the systematic and logical relationships among sounds. With this perception and practice, his auditory skills improve. The sounds must be carefully selected in order for him to make order out of chaos. But the sounds used for practice on discrimination do not always easily fit into the ordinary words and sentences that would help him communicate with his family and friends. The patient needs to use and understand words and phrases. He needs to begin work on reading and writing concurrently with work on sound recognition, discrimination, and production.

Patients with auditory processing involvement experience much the same difficulty in reading and writing as they do in speaking. Luria says:[50]

> Such patients cannot distinguish the necessary acoustic content of a word, they begin to confuse similarly sounding phonemes and they can no longer analyze complex combinations of sounds. The patient is able to copy and he is able to write familiar words such as his name and address. These words do not require acoustic analysis and have become a stable motor stereotype. [p. 140]

For these patients, the word 'limes' may sound like 'lines' or 'lions.' They rarely notice their errors, even when errors are pointed out to them. They receive few or no cues from spelling the word aloud. Until the patient attains more discrimination skill, words and phrases and sentences selected for reading and writing should contain only the sounds worked on in therapy. This means that the therapist must take the time to write or carefully select the materials to use for reading aloud and for comprehension. Patients, however, gain sounds quickly and after three to six weeks, depending upon the severity of the auditory involvement, they become able to handle more complex words for reading and writing tasks.

Patients who have had some practice on auditory discrimination as described above, may develop reading skills which are superior to their skills in auditory comprehension because of the cues obtained from the printed words. The formulation of short sentences, grouped according to sentence pattern, may contribute to a patient's understanding of the structure and content of sentences he might wish to use. For example, lists of sentences which focus on a particular linguistic structure might be developed. One list might include sentences like:

The sky is blue, the grass is green, the door is open.

Another list might include:

The stores are open, the books are heavy, the days are long.

Other examples are:

I am hungry, I am tired, I am thirsty; it is raining, it is snowing, it is getting late.

Occasionally, patients benefit from control of the lexicon—the systematic addition of concrete, abstract and proper nouns, of descriptive adjectives and verbs, of definite and indefinite articles, of the copula 'be' of pronouns, of conjunctions, of the negative 'not', and of interrogatives.[37, 51-54]

Spontaneous Speech

The LCT is designed to be an adjunct to more traditional therapy methods and whatever variations individual therapists might wish to use are encouraged. It is not so much the content as it is the structure of the approach that makes it successful. In addition to the suggestions described above, the therapist should encourage the patient to use spontaneously the words, phrases, and sentences which he has come to understand, read, write, and speak. Often, patients do not need specific and prolonged work on sentences. The foundation that has been laid in therapy is sufficient for them to build upon, and they spontaneously begin using a variety of sentence constructions. There are some patients who have particular difficulty with nouns, with verb forms, or with other parts of speech. These patients seem unable to incorporate these constructions into their spontaneous speech even with the use of the exercises outlined above.

If patients have progressed through the preceding steps, they are able to read and repeat some simple sentences. One way of assisting them with categorization is to provide them with a series of appropriate pictures and a chart with one sentence pattern illustrated several times. For example, for a picture in which a young boy has locked himself in the bathroom and is crying while his family tries different methods of unlocking the door, the sentences might be:

Pattern 1:	Noun	Verb	Adjective
	The bathtub	is	full.
	The door	is	locked.
	The sink	is	white.

The patient is directed to talk about the picture and/or write several descriptive sentences like the ones on the chart. Other pictures are presented and the patient proceeds with the same task. Several variations of the pattern may be made. For example:

Pattern 2:	Pronoun	Verb	Noun
	There	is	a boy.
	There	is	a shower.
	There	is	a rug.
	He	is	a boy.
	She	is	a mother.
	He	is	a father.
	It	is	a rug.

Other patterns may be introduced after the patient is able to describe the pictures within the sentence frameworks listed above. For example, the following variations:

The father	tries	the key.
The boy	washes	his face.
The boat	sinks	in the water.
The boy	stands	on the chair.
The mother	yells	at the boy.

There are other sentence structures that can be used, and sentences may be constructed according to different criteria. Naeser[39] used the same kind of structured approach in working with aphasic patients, but she did not use the same sentence patterns. She worked separately with transitive and intransitive verbs, and her results suggested that patients receiving this approach improved at a faster rate than those who did not. She also concluded that this technique is most beneficial to patients with posterior aphasia.

One problem sometimes encountered is that patients may have difficulty limiting their responses to only the ones required. When this happens, it can be helpful to construct simple sentences that answer the questions 'what', 'when', 'where', 'why', and 'how'. Pictures might be presented with the question, 'Who is doing what?' and the patient admonished to limit his response to the precise answer. This tends to minimize extraneous remarks, and offers the patient either a firm sentence pattern to follow or the opportunity to proceed with sentence patterns of his own construction.

COMMENTS

Several comments based on research, experience, and common sense should be directed to the issue of the importance of diagnosing auditory processing disorders, and the treatment of severe language disturbance. Diagnosis results when the subtle aspects of difficulties in auditory processing can be separated from the language problem, and then identified. Currently, not enough is known about the relationship between language and auditory processing to allow for an easy, step by step method of identifying specific auditory processing disorders in aphasic patients. For mildly involved patients, it may not be necessary because they appear to respond well to the more traditional language therapy techniques. Moderately involved patients seem to progress more rapidly in therapy when rigid control of auditory input is utilized with the more traditional therapy techniques. For the large number of patients who are more severely involved, rigid control of auditory input seems essential. To assist in the process of identifying auditory processing disorders, the answers to the following questions can be of assistance:

Are the mistakes similar in sound to the target word?
Are short words missed?
Is performance disproportionately better on visual than on auditory tasks?
Is there an on-off effect?
Do multiple repetitions of the stimuli increase accuracy of responses?
Are single sounds discriminated?
Can the patient follow verbal directions?
Can the patient comprehend the main idea of a short sentence or paragraph?

The answers to these questions can provide a basis for developing a therapy plan that works despite the lack of a definitive theoretic description of the auditory processing disorder.

Factors such as age, general health, economics, motivation, and the availability of therapy should be considered in the determination of therapy plans; it is not always practical or reasonable to provide therapy for a particular patient. Therapy, based on as thorough an understanding as possible of the nature of the deficit, can help the patient's total recovery. Structured approaches similar to the LCT have been used successfully.[39, 55] For a patient who has regained no language function in any modality six months after the stroke, the addition of 20 phrases and sentences to his life, with the Melodic Intonation Therapy technique,[34] for example, makes a joyful difference to him and his family. For a patient considered to have global aphasia three months after his stroke, but reclassified three months later as having a severe auditory processing disorder and apraxia, long-term therapy (in this case, three years) using the LCT made the difference between vegetating in front of a television set and returning, part time, to a company for which he had worked prior to the stroke. For these patients, the number of hours spent in therapy was very small compared to what the results contributed to their quality of life.

Within the framework of what we know is possible, rehabilitation of language function can occur in many more patients than is currently considered practical.

REFERENCES

1. Johnston KL: Longitudinal study of language test performance by patients with occlusive lesions (unpublished paper). NINCDS, NIH, Cerebrovascular Clinical Research Center Grant, NS-03364, 1962–1978
2. Rubens AB, Ramirez-Lassepas M, Johnston KL: Unpublished data, 1974
3. Rochford G: Are jargon dysphasics dysphasic? Br J Disord Commun 9:35–44, 1974

4. Needham LS, Swisher LP: A comparison of three tests of auditory comprehension for adult aphasics. J Speech Hearing Dis 37:123–131, 1972
5. Duffy RJ, Ulrich S: A comparison of impairments in verbal comprehension, speech reading and writing in adult aphasics. J Speech Hearing Dis 41:110–119, 1976
6. Schuell H: Minnesota Test for Differential Diagnosis of Aphasia (rev ed). Minneapolis, University of Minnesota Press, 1972
7. Goodglass H, Kaplan E: The Assessment of Aphasia and Related Disorders. Philadelphia, Lea and Febiger, 1972
8. Spreen O, Benton AL: Neurosensory Center Comprehensive Examination for Aphasia (rev ed). Victoria, British Columbia, University of Victoria, 1969
9. Porch BE: Porch Index of Communicative Ability (rev ed). Palo Alto, Consulting Psychologists Press, 1971
10. Ammons RB, Ammons HS: Full Range Picture Vocabulary Test. Missoula, Montana, Psychological Test Specialists, 1948
11. Dunn LM: Peabody Picture Vocabulary Test. Circle Pines, Minnesota, American Guidance Service, 1959, 1965
12. Jastak J, Jastak SR: Wide Range Achievement Test (rev ed). Austin, Guidance Testing Associates, 1965
13. Gates AI, MacGinitie WH: Gates-MacGinitie Reading Tests. New York, Teachers College Press, 1965
14. Wepman J: Wepman Test of Auditory Discrimination. Chicago, Language Research Associates, 1973
15. DeRenzi E, Vignolo LA: The Token Test: A sensitive test to detect receptive disturbances in aphasics. Brain 85:665–678, 1962
16. Baker HR, Leland B: Detroit Tests of Learning Aptitude. Indianapolis, Bobbs-Merrill, 1968
17. Kirk SA, McCarthy JJ, Kirk WD: Illinois Test of Pyscholinguistic Abilities (rev ed). Urbana, University of Illinois Press, 1975
18. Luria AR: Higher Cortical Functions in Man. New York, Basic Books, 1966, p 187
19. Darley FL, Aronson AE, Brown JE: Motor Speech Disorders. Philadelphia, W. B. Saunders, 1975
20. Sands ES, Freeman FJ, Harris KS: Progressive changes in articulatory patterns in verbal apraxia: A longitudinal case study. Brain Lang 6:97–105, 1978
21. Schuell H: Differential Diagnosis. Lecture, October, 1965
22. Johns DF, Darley FL: Phonemic variability in apraxia of speech. J Speech Hearing Res 13:556–583, 1970
23. Macmahon MKC: Modern linguistics and aphasia. Br J Disord Commun 7:54–63, 1972
24. Johnston KL: Differences among examiners in the classification of types of aphasia (unpublished paper). NINCDS, NIH, Cerebrovascular Clinical Research Center Grant, NS-03364, 1962–1978
25. Eisenson J: Adult Aphasia: Assessment and Treatment. New York, Appleton-Century-Crofts, 1973
26. Smith A: Diagnosis, intelligence and rehabilitation of chronic aphasics: A final report. Ann Arbor, University of Michigan Department of Physical Medicine and Rehabilitation, 1972
27. Darley FL: Treatment of acquired aphasia, in Friedlander WJ (ed): Advances in Neurology, vol. 7. New York, Raven Press, 1975, pp111–145
28. Culton GL: Spontaneous recovery from aphasia. J Speech Hearing Res. 12:825–832, 1969
29. Sarno MT, Levita E: Natural course of recovery in severe aphasia. Arch Phys Med 52: 175–179, 1971
30. Kertesz A, McCabe P: Recovery patterns and prognosis in aphasia. Brain 100:1–18, 1977

31. Eisenson J: Language rehabilitation of aphasic adults: A review of some issues as to the state of the art, in Sullivan M, Kommers MS (eds): Rationale for Adult Aphasia Therapy. Omaha, University of Nebraska Medical Center, 1976, pp1–28
32. Beyn ES: Basic principles of restorative therapy on speech in aphasia. Bibl Psychiatry Neurol 139:174–188, 1969
33. Language Master Cards. Bell and Howell, Chicago
34. Helm N: Melodic Intonation Therapy Workshop. Courage Center, Golden Valley, Minnesota, November 1-2, 1974. Co-sponsored by the Aphasia Center, Hennepin County Medical Center; Department of Communication Disorders, University of Minnesota; Aphasia Section, Minneapolis Veterans Administration Hospital
35. Caplan LR: Variability of perceptual function: The sensory cortex as a "categorizer" and "deducer." Brain Lang 6:1–13, 1978
36. Jakobson R: Toward a linguistic classification of aphasic impairments, in Goodglass H, Blumstein S (eds): Psycholinguistics and Aphasia. Baltimore, Johns Hopkins University Press, 1973, pp29–47
37. Ulatowska HK, Richardson SH: A longitudinal study of an adult with aphasia: Considerations for research and therapy. Brain Lang 1:151–166, 1974
38. Hatfield FM: Looking for help from linguistics. Br J Disord Commun 7:64–81, 1972
39. Naeser MA: A structured approach teaching aphasics basic sentence types. Br J Disord Commun 10:70–76, 1975
40. Parker F: Distinctive features in speech pathology: Phonology or phonemics? J Speech Hearing Dis 41:23–39, 1976
41. Luria AR: Restoration of Function After Brain Injury (Eng trans). New York, Macmillan, 1963
42. Lerner JW: Children with Learning Disabilities. Boston, Houghton Mifflin, 1976, pp241–243
43. Keller E: Parameters for vowel substitutions in Broca's aphasia. Brain Lang 5:265–285, 1978
44. Blumstein SE: The use and theoretical implications of the dichotic technique for investigating distinctive features. Brain Lang 1:337–350, 1974
45. Tallal P, Piercy M: Developmental aphasia: The perception of brief vowels and extended stop consonants. Neuropsychologia 13:69–74, 1975
46. Trost JE, Canter GJ: Apraxia of speech in patients with Broca's aphasia: A study of phoneme production accuracy and error patterns. Brain Lang 1:63–79, 1974
47. Studdert-Kennedy M, Shankweiler D: Hemispheric specialization for speech perception. J Acoust Soc Am 48:579–594, 1970
48. Zlatin MA, Koenigsknecht RA: Development of the voicing contrast: Perception of stop consonants. J Speech Hearing Res 18:541–553, 1975
49. Dabul B, Bollier B: Therapeutic approaches to apraxia. J Speech Hearing Dis 41:268–276, 1976
50. Luria AR: The Working Brain. New York, Basic Books, 1973, p140
51. Mihăilescu L, Weigh I, Weigl E, Kreindler A: Performance in aphasics at conceptual and operational words used single or within syntagms. Rev Roum Neurol 9:181–195, 1972
52. Kreindler A, Mihăilescu L, Weigh I: Aphasic performance to syntagms. Rev Roum Neurol 11:227–242, 1974
53. Gardner H, Zurif E: Bee but not be: Oral reading of single words in aphasia and alexia. Neuropsychologia 13:181–190, 1975
54. Gardner H: The contribution of operativity to naming capacity in aphasic patients. Neuropsychologia 11:213–220, 1973
55. Harris C: Auditory processing disability: Sixteen months of treatment, in Andrews JR,

Burns MS (Eds): Selected Papers in Language and Phonology, vol. II. Evanston, Institute for Continuing Professional Education, 1977, pp1–6

56. Wertz RT: Appraisal and diagnosis in aphasia: Evaluating the effects of treatment, in Sullivan M, Kommers MS (eds): Rationale for Adult Aphasia Therapy. Omaha, University of Nebraska Medical Center, 1976, pp44–96

Isabelle Y. Liberman, Donald Shankweiler,
Linda Camp, Benita Blachman,
and Michele Werfelman

10

Steps Toward Literacy: A Linguistic Approach*

The reading curricula commonly used in our schools appear to us not to take advantage of an important and readily available body of knowledge about the relationship between reading and the spoken language. That is unfortunate, if, as we believe, much of that knowledge might be put to good use in the prevention of reading failure. In the first section of this chapter, we will, by way of background, review some relevant information, particularly that which concerns the way in which an orthography transcribes the language. We will also describe associated research results, together with the more general view of the reading process that they support. In the second section, we will develop the implications for reading instruction.

We should emphasize that we do not intend to present a reading curriculum with all the detail that such an undertaking would require. What we can offer are guidelines for early reading instruction that are consistent with what is known about linguistic factors in reading, including mainly that research in which we have a special interest.

---

*This chapter is adapted from a report prepared for the *Working Group on Learning Failure and Unused Learning Potential* for the President's Commission on Mental Health, Washington, D.C. November 1, 1977. Some of the material in this report has also appeared in Resnick L, Weaver P (eds): Theory and Practice of Early Reading, Vol. 2. Hillsdale, New Jersey, Erlbaum Associates, 1979.

SPEECH, THE ALPHABET, AND LEARNING TO READ

Reading and the Spoken Language

We assume at the outset that reading is intimately related to and, indeed, dependent on speech. We are led to this assumption by several observations that seem obvious and compelling.[1, 2] First, speech and reading both have to do with language: speech is language for the ear, while reading is language for the eye. But speech is unquestionably the primary language system while reading is secondary. Speech is universal, while reading is rare among many of the world's peoples. Speech was first in the evolution of man, while reading was second and a comparatively recent development in man's history. Speech is also first in the history of the individual while reading comes second. Speech is, moreover, remarkably easy for humans to acquire. Infants are already listening discriminatively to speech by the age of one month,[3] and most two-year-olds are already beginning to speak intelligibly. Speech apparently requires little tuition, only an input of linguistic data and an opportunity to interact with those data. In contrast, reading is difficult and ordinarily is not acquired unless taught.

The second observation that leads to the assumption that reading is dependent on speech has to do with the nature of the writing system. We all know that human language is distinguished from other communication systems by the fact that it is phonemic. That is, all human languages are composed of commutable segments that have no meaning in themselves. These segments, called phonemes, can be transmitted either by ear or by eye—that is, by spoken or written language. An alphabetic writing system, such as English, is a more or less accurate representation of the phonologic structure of the spoken language; it is not, as some educators seem to believe, a symbol system keyed directly to meaning.

Finally, evidence to support the contention that speech is an essential foundation for the acquisition of reading is seen in the remarkably poor reading achievement of the congenitally deaf. We know that these children, who are blocked in the acquisition of speech, do not readily learn to read even though they have complete access to the printed word through the visual channel.[4]

In summary, reading is parasitic on speech and cannot be reasonably considered apart from speech.[5] If reading and speech are so closely linked, it is surely unparsimonious to imagine a completely parallel language understanding system for reading that borrows nothing from the primary speech system. We assume, therefore, that the reading process must necessarily tie in with the speech system at some point. The way in which this is done will depend on the nature of the writing system.

Reading and the Writing System

How does the nature of the writing system affect the task of reading acquisition? Before we can answer that question, we must first consider in what ways the spoken language can be represented by its written counterpart. To write a language, one must decide which of its several kinds and sizes of segments should be represented.[6] The choice of kind arises from the fact that all languages have a dual structure—segments that have meaning and segments that do not. Each kind of segment offers its own set of options in size. For example, meaningful segments can be as long as sentences or as short as words. Among the meaningless segments, the most likely candidates for a writing system are syllables and phonemes, the latter being the shortest segments of all.

THE HISTORICAL DEVELOPMENT OF WRITING

In the historical development of writing, systems that used meaningful units came first.[7, 8] Some were historically related; others developed independently. Something like the word was the segment most commonly represented. The Chinese ideographic characters and the kanji characters of Japanese are present-day examples of this method. In these writing systems, a single character or symbol denotes a word.

Writing systems based on meaningless units are a more recent development. Among these, the segment size that was represented in all the earliest systems was the syllable. In these writing systems, as in the present-day kana part of Japanese, a single character denotes a syllable ('ba, be, bi, bu, ga, ge, gi, gu', for example). An alphabet, representing segments of phonemic size ('b', 'a', 't', for example), was developed much later. It is clear, moreover, that the alphabet developed historically out of a syllabary and, furthermore, that this important development, quite unlike the others, occurred only once. All subsequent alphabets are derivations of the original one invented by a Phoenician trader.

ABSTRACTING THE UNIT TO BE REPRESENTED

Writing systems, as we have noted, can represent the spoken language by segments of different kinds and sizes. However, whatever the kind or the size of the segment, it is obvious that the inventor of the writing system must first have succeeded in consciously abstracting that unit from the acoustic stream of speech. What does the history of writing systems tell us about this? As we have pointed out, writing systems based on meaningless units, the syllables and phonemes, were late developments in the history of written languages. The alphabetic system, which requires the abstraction of the phonemic unit of speech, was the last to appear; it evolved from a syllabary and, in contrast to other systems, was apparently invented only once.

It seems reasonable to suppose that this historical progression from word to syllable to phoneme might reflect the ease (or difficulty) of abstracting segments of a particular type from the speech stream.[9] From this it would follow that the order of difficulty of segmentation would be: the word, the syllable and, hardest of all, the phoneme. More to the point of this paper, we should suppose that for the young child learning to read, there might be the same order of difficulty. That is, the child learning to read in an alphabetic system may be faced with the most difficult level of analysis in the early stages of attaining literacy. In the next section, we will explore this question in more detail.

Reading Acquisition and the Alphabet

In languages that are written alphabetically, the unit characters or letters are keyed to the phonologic structure of speech. We are aware that the mapping from written symbols to phonemes is more nearly one-to-one in some alphabetic languages, such as Finnish and Serbo-Croatian, than in English. The many departures from one-to-one mapping makes English difficult to spell, and probably more difficult to learn to read, than is the case in languages whose alphabetic writing systems have a more regular structure. Nonetheless, it is important to underscore the fact that English spelling, in common with other orthographies that employ an alphabet, is, for all its peculiarities, a cipher on the phonemes of the language.[2]

THE ADVANTAGES OF THE ALPHABET AND AN ANALYTIC STRATEGY

The child's fundamental task in learning to read is to construct a link between speech and the alphabetic cipher. It is appropriate at this point to remind ourselves of the benefits that alphabets confer.[10, 11] A unique advantage of an alphabetic system is that each new word does not have to be memorized, as if it were an ideographic character, before it can be read. That is, given a word that is already in his spoken language, the reader can apprehend the word without specific instruction, although he may never have seen it before in print. Or, given a word that he has never before seen or heard, he can closely approximate its spoken form until its meaning can be inferred from context or discovered later by asking someone about it. The letters, by functioning however roughly as surrogates for phonemes, enable users of the alphabet to gain immediate access to all items in a vast word store by means of a highly economical set of symbols.

The savings may be had, however, only by the user who knows how the alphabet works. As in all complex cognitive skills, alternative strategies are possible. The very diversity of the orthographies that have developed during the course of the evolution of writing is testimony to the flexibility of the perceptual apparatus. It is, of course, possible to read words written by an alphabet as though they were ideographs. Many children undoubtedly begin reading acquisition in this way.

THE NEED FOR EXPLICIT AWARENESS OF THE PHONEMIC LEVEL

The unique advantages of the alphabet, however, are closed to the child who cannot use it analytically. Although alphabetically written words can be treated as ideographs, using such a strategy will not help the child to apprehend new words. In order to make the alphabet work for them, children have to be able to make an explicit analysis of the phonemic segments of the spoken language. First, they must realize that speech can be segmented into phonemes, and they must know the number of phonemes the words in their vocabulary contain and the order in which they occur. Second, they must know that the letter symbols represent phonemes and not syllables or some other unit of speech. This sort of explicit awareness of the phonemic properties of speech is a precondition for understanding the alphabetic principle.

When we speak of explicit knowledge of the segments in the spoken message, we wish to make it very clear that something more is involved than the ordinary competence required in language use. That is to say, a person may be a completely adequate speaker-hearer of his language without having any awareness that the spoken word 'bet' contains three phoneme segments, and 'best' contains four. The immediate recognition of these as different words, in the absence of the ability to indicate that 's' is the unshared segment, is an example of what Polanyi[12] has called "tacit knowledge." Such knowledge is sufficient for comprehension of the spoken message. Writing and reading, on the other hand, demand an additional analytic capability, as will be pointed out later in some detail.

THE DIFFICULTY OF EXPLICIT AWARENESS OF PHONEME SEGMENTATION

There are several lines of indirect evidence which suggest that this needed awareness of the structure of the spoken word is not readily attainable by the child. The first, the historical development of writing systems, has already been discussed. Another relevant finding is that children with reading disabilities often have difficulties even with spoken language when they are required to perform tasks demanding some degree of conscious segmentation of phonemic structure. For example, these children are often reported to be deficient in rhyming, in recognizing that two different monosyllables may share the same first (or last) phonemic segment,[13] and according to recent research,[14] in speaking Pig Latin, which demands a conscious shift of the initial phonemic segment to the final position in the word.

A third line of evidence is provided by the behavior of reading disabled children as observed by teachers who have worked with them.[15] These children will demonstrate, as we have suggested earlier, that they can readily recover the phonemic segments in the ordinary course of speaking and listening. That is, they can respond appropriately to spoken words and to the objects to which they refer. Moreover, they can approximate the letter-to-sound correspondences. For example, if they are asked to give the sound of the letter *b*, they will say "bŭh". For the letter *a*, they will say "ă" (although this may give them more trouble, as we will discuss later). For the sound of the letter *t*, they will say "tŭh." But if they are shown the printed word *bat*, and asked to read it, they may give any one of a variety of incorrect responses that begin with the letter *b*, but otherwise bear little relation to the original word. If they are pressed to try to "sound out" the word, or otherwise to use what they know about the letter-to-sound correspondences, they are likely to produce "bŭhătŭh." At that point, they may be urged by the teacher to "say it faster," to "put the sounds together," or, in the phrase commonly used, to "blend it." But no matter how fast they produce those sounds or how desperately they try to put them together, they often produce the nonword "bŭhătŭh", containing five phonemic segments, and not the word 'bat', which has only three. Somehow they cannot relate the three letters of the printed word to the three phonemic segments of the spoken word. It is as if they were not aware of the fact that the monosyllabic spoken word has three segments.[9]

AN EXPLANATION FOR THE DIFFICULTY OF ABSTRACTING PHONEMIC SEGMENTS

Why should it be so difficult for the child to become explicitly aware of phonemic segmentation? If, as has often been supposed, the sounds of speech bore a simple one-to-one relationship to the phonemic structure of the language, just as the letters do (at least in the orthographically regular case), it would indeed be hard to see why phonemic analysis should pose special problems. That is, if there were in the word 'bat' three acoustic segments—one for each of the three phonemes—the segmentation of the word that is represented by its spelling would be readily apparent.

However, extensive research in speech perception has shown that the segmentation of the acoustic signal does not correspond directly or in any easily determined way to the segmentation at the phonemic level.[5, 16, 17] Moreover, this lack of correspondence does not arise because the sounds of the phonemes are merely linked together, as are the letters of the alphabet in cursive writing (or as may be implied by the reading teacher who urges the child to blend "bŭhătŭh" into a word that he knows). Instead, the phonemic segments are encoded or merged at the acoustic level into essentially unitary sounds of approximately syllabic dimensions. In the case of 'bat', for example, the initial and final consonants are folded into the medial vowel, so that information about the successive segments of the word is transmitted more or less simultaneously on the same parts of the sound.[18] In exactly that sense, the syllable, 'bat', which has three phonemic segments, has but one acoustic segment in which the phonemes are merged.[9]

The merging of phonemes in the speech stream complicates the process of discovery of the phonemic structure of speech for the would-be reader. However, we should emphasize again that the child who finds it difficult to make explicit the phonemic segmentation of his speech need not have any problems at all with speaking and listening. Children generally distinguish (or identify) words like 'bad' and 'bag', which differ in only one phonemic segment. Indeed, there is evidence that infants at one month of age discriminate sounds categorically.[3] (Chapter 3). The child has no difficulty speaking and listening to speech, because segmentation of the largely continuous acoustic signal is done automatically by operations about which he is not conscious.* In order to speak and listen, the child need have no more conscious awareness of phonemic structure than he has of syntactic structure. In that connection, we all know that a child can speak grammatical sentences without being able to explicate their structure. Similarly, he can readily distinguish 'bad' from 'bag' without being able to analyze the underlying phonemic structure—that is, without an explicit understanding of the fact that each of these utterances consists of three segments and that the difference between them lies wholly in the third segment. But reading, unlike speech, does require a more explicit analysis if the advantages of an alphabet are to be realized.[10, 11]

The encoded nature of phonemes has another consequence that contributes to the difficulty in learning to read analytically; it is impossible to read by sounding out the letters one by one. In the example of 'bag', used above, reading letter by letter gives not "bag", but "bŭhăgŭh." In order to learn to read analytically, one must achieve something altogether different: one must discover how many of the letter segments must be taken into account simultaneously in order to arrive at the correct phonetic rendition. In the case of the word 'bag', there is reason to believe that the number would be three. But, in fact, there is no simple rule for arriving at that number, and we suspect that learning to group the letters for the purpose of proper phonetic recoding is one of the really significant skills a reader must acquire. Even in languages like Finnish and Spanish, in which the writing system closely approximates a one-to-one correspondence between letters and phonemes, reading cannot be a simple matter of association between alphabetic character and spoken sound. In order to recover the spoken form, the reader must chunk all the letters that represent the phonemic segments encoded into each syllable. In the case of reading a word in isolation, the coding unit is probably the syllable.[10, 11]

*This may not be the case for some children who have difficulty acquiring speech and language. In these cases, it may be necessary to make the structure explicit to facilitate learning of the spoken language. See Chapter 7.

THE RELATIVE EASE OF SYLLABIC ANALYSIS

If it is now apparent why explicit segmentation into phonemes might be difficult, it is still reasonable to ask why syllables should be easier.[9] A plausible answer is not hard to find. As we noted earlier, the consonant segments of the phonemic message are typically folded, at the acoustic level, into the vowel. The result is that there is no acoustic criterion by which the phonemic segments are dependably marked. However, every syllable that is formed in this way contains a vocalic nucleus and, therefore, a peak of acoustic energy. These energy peaks provide audible cues that correspond to the syllable centers.[19] Though such auditory cues could not in themselves help a listener to define exact syllable boundaries, they should make it easy for him to discover how many syllables there are and, in that sense, to do explicit syllabic segmentation.

If syllabic segmentation is easier, we then have an explanation for the assertion that the Japanese kana is readily mastered.[20] The kana is one of the two Japanese writing systems, and is approximately a syllabary. Most of the graphic symbols in the kana represent a syllable, as we have said. There are separate symbols for ba, be, bi, bu, ga, ge, gi, gu, and so on. Given the open syllable (CV) structure of the Japanese spoken language, the child, therefore, rarely needs to go below the level of the syllable in order to master the writing system. Similarly, an orthography in which each character represents a word (as is the case in Chinese ideographs or in the closely related Japanese kanji) should also be easier for the beginning reader, at least sparing him the particular difficulties that arise in mastering the more analytic alphabetic system. Indirect evidence of the special burden imposed on the beginning reader by an alphabetic script can be found in the relative ease with which reading-disabled children learn kanji-like representations of language while they are unable to break the alphabetic cipher.[21]

THE DEVELOPMENTAL PROGRESSION OF SEGMENTAL ANALYSIS

There is a growing body of empirical evidence that demonstrates more directly that phonemic segmentation is harder than syllabic segmentation, and that the ability to do it develops later.[6, 22-24] These findings are typified by a recent investigation by our research group.[6] The point of our study was to determine how well children in nursery school, kindergarten, and first grade (four-, five-, and six-year-olds) can identify the number of phonemic segments in spoken utterances, and how this compares with their ability to deal similarly with syllables. The procedure was in the form of a game that required the child to indicate, by tapping a wooden dowel on the table, the number (from 1 to 3) of the segments (phonemes in one group, syllables in the other) in a list of test utterances.

At age four, none of the children could segment by phoneme, whereas nearly half could segment by syllable. The ability to carry out phoneme segmentation successfully did not appear until age five, and then it was demonstrated by less than one-fifth of the children. In contrast, almost half of the children at that age could segment syllabically. Even at age six, only 70 percent succeeded in phoneme segmentation, while 90 percent were successful in the syllable task.

SEGMENTATION ABILITY AND READING SKILL

The difficulty of phoneme segmentation and its possible importance as an entry behavior for reading acquisition has been affirmed by many investigators besides ourselves.[14, 24-31] We explored this question directly by measuring the reading achievement of the children who had taken part in our experiment on phoneme segmentation. We tested our first graders at the beginning of their second school year and found that half of the children in the lowest third of the class in reading achievement had failed the segmentation task the previous June. On the other hand, there were no failures in phoneme segmentation among children who scored in the top third of the class in reading ability.[6]

A number of new studies now confirm these results.[32-35] Despite widely varying school populations (from black disadvantaged to white middle-class school children) and quite diverse experimental procedures, each of these studies shows a high and significant correlation between success in phoneme segmentation and early reading ability. All of these studies suggest that the ability to analyze speech phonemically is indeed relevant to success or failure in learning to read. The results lend encouragement to the hypothesis that segmentation ability may be critically associated with reading acquisition.*

THE PATTERN OF READING ERRORS AS INDICATORS OF PROBLEMS IN READING ACQUISITION

We have suggested that a lack of awareness of phonemic segmentation may be one serious roadblock to reading acquisition. There are data from the analysis of children's reading errors that appear to provide additional indirect evidence for this view. It seemed to us[9] that if a child's chief problem in reading is that he cannot make explicit the phonemic structure of the language, he might be expected to show success in identifying the initial letter of words (requiring no further analysis of the syllable), and relatively poor performance beyond that point. If all he knows are the letter-to-sound corre-

*In a recent study, it was reported that adult illiterates had difficulty in carrying out phonemic segmentation of spoken words, whereas others from the same community who had learned to read as adults were able to perform segmentation tasks.[55] These findings suggest that literacy training, and not maturation alone, may be critical for the development of conscious awareness of phonemic structure.

spondences and that he must proceed from left to right, he might in the case of 'bat', for example, simply pronounce the phoneme corresponding to the first letter, and then search his lexicon for a word beginning with that phoneme. Of course, what he needs to do instead is to search his lexicon for a word that has three phonemic segments corresponding to the letter segments in the printed word. However, if he does not know that the words in his lexicon have segments or if he finds phonemic segmentation difficult, he will not be able to map the letters to the segments in those words. By this reasoning, his errors on the final consonants in words should be greater than those on the initial consonants.

That is precisely what we found in a series of experiments on the reading of monosyllabic words by second, third, and fourth graders.[9, 36, 37] There was indeed a progression of difficulty related to the position of the segment in the word with the final consonants being misread twice as frequently as the initial consonants. Similar findings have been reported by other investigators who examined error patterns in the reading of connected text.[38, 39]

VOWEL ORTHOGRAPHY AS ANOTHER SOURCE OF DIFFICULTY

So far we have presented several lines of evidence suggesting that the explicit analysis of phoneme segmentation is a hard and unnatural task that may be an important source of difficulty for the child learning to read. But it is certainly not the only serious barrier. The error pattern for reading vowels provides a case in point.[11] It is well established that in English vowels elicit many more errors than consonants.[11, 13, 39, 40] In the reading errors study described above, for example, the vowel errors were roughly twice as frequent as the overall consonant errors.

Why should the error rate for reading vowels be so much higher than that for consonants? It might be simply because of the embedded medial position of the vowel in the words used to test reading. To check on this possibility, we devised a new reading test consisting of equal numbers of words containing vowels in the initial, medial, and final positions. It was found that the overall rate of vowel errors continued to be about twice that of consonant errors, regardless of vowel position in words.

There are two reasons for suspecting that vowel errors may reflect something more than the segmentation problems we discussed in relation to consonant errors. First, as we have seen, the child can apparently count syllables fairly well, and the vowel nucleus stands out in the spoken word as a major element that can be identified in the syllable. A second, and perhaps more interesting reason, can be seen from further examination of the error patterns. In the case of consonants, errors tend to pile up in the final position. We have taken this to be indirect evidence that the child is having segmentation problems. Vowel errors, on the other hand, are different. In our error studies, there was no significant difference in error rate for vowels whether they occurred in the initial, medial, or final position. Moreover, the error rate of vowels in both initial and final positions continued to be significantly higher when compared with consonant errors in corresponding positions. In English, there is clearly no position effect evident in vowel errors; they are simply difficult in all positions. Thus, the vowel problem certainly cannot be entirely attributed to segmentation difficulties.

We suspect that the errors elicited by consonants and those elicited by vowels are quite different in their origins. In the case of consonants, the child has little trouble learning the spelling-to-sound correspondences. Furthermore, orthographic complexity makes no appreciable difference to the position effect of consonants. The child's error pattern there arises mainly from the fact that he cannot map the segmentation of the printed word to the segmentation of the spoken word.

The extra difficulties attendant upon the vowels are probably due in part to the obvious orthographic complexities of the spelling-to-sound correspondence for vowels,* but also partly to the continuous and fluid nature of vowel perception.[5, 18] Although it stands out wherever it occurs in speech, the vowel can be spelled in many ways in the English writing system, and is less categorically perceived than the consonants. That is, not only is there a many-to-one mapping of spelling-to-sound (*a* may have the sound 'ă' as in 'cat' or 'a' as in 'baby'), but also there is the continuous nature of vowel perception, which makes the sound correspondences of single vowel letters harder to code and to maintain in memory. We have argued that because of the continuous nature of their perception, vowels tend to be somewhat indefinite phonologic entities.[37] This is also illustrated by the major part they play in the variations among dialects, and the persistence of allophones within a geographic locality. By this reasoning, it could be that the less strongly categorical nature of vowel perception may itself be one cause of the complex orthography for vowels, and at least one reason why multiple representations of vowels are tolerated.

Although we believe that it is of interest to investigate the causes of vowel errors, we recognize that the vowel may be less important in the process of reading acquisition than would first appear. It could be argued that if the child's segmentation problems were corrected, his difficulties with

*In this connection, it is of interest to report that though the position effect in the consonant error pattern has been replicated in the reading of Serbo-Croatian words, the vowel error rate did not exceed the consonant rate; indeed, it was significantly less. Serbo-Croatian differs from English in two respects that are relevant here—the vowel set is limited to five vowels and the written language is orthographically extremely regular.[56]

vowels would not be a serious barrier to reading acquisition. Consonants carry most of the information load. If the child knew how many consonants there were and their sequence in the spoken word, an incorrect rendition of the vowel sound would be fairly easily corrected in the context. Getting only the vowel correct, without a proper analysis of the phonemic sequence of the word, would be of less benefit to him.

Theoretical Summary

We believe that the priority of spoken language and the recognition of how reading and writing are derived from it are the starting points for any understanding of writing systems and their acquisition. Reading presents special problems for the perceiver; these problems reflect the manner in which the writing system makes contact with the primary speech system. In the case of English, the ties between the language and its spelling are based in part at least on the phonemic structure. Therefore, it is particularly appropriate to direct the child's attention to the phonemic level of language because the phonemic correspondences are the entry points to any alphabetic writing system.

In order to learn to read an alphabetically written language, the child must have the ability to make explicit the segmentation of his own speech, particularly at the level of the phoneme. Data were presented that indicate that explicit awareness of the phonemic structure is difficult to attain; this is in contrast to the tacit appreciation of phonemic contrasts reflected in ordinary language use. We and others have shown that the capacity to abstract the phonemic segment is lacking in many children when they start to learn to read, and may contribute to reading failure. The vowel orthography poses other, additional problems.

The relationships between speech and reading are both intimate and subtle. It would seem appropriate for the early instruction in reading to take these factors into account if the child is to master an alphabetically written language.

SPEECH, THE ALPHABET, AND TEACHING TO READ

It has become fashionable to say that very little is known about how to teach reading, and that the teacher makes a greater difference than the method. We would agree that the flexibility and wisdom teachers show in adapting existing curricula to meet individual differences, as well as their ability to recognize the necessity for doing so, will always be important variables in the success of any instructional procedure. However, we would also maintain that the little we do know about reading is often not reflected in reading curricula. If it were, even the less creative teacher might be more successful, and the proportion of children resistant to reading instruction might be decreased.[2]

To take a very basic example, consider what we know about our writing system—namely, that it is alphabetic and not ideographic. From this, it follows that instructional procedures should inform the child from the very beginning that the printed word is a model of the ordered string of component phonemes in the spoken word and their particular succession. Conversely, it would follow that the instruction should not, as it often does, mislead the child into assuming that the printed word is an ideographic symbol—a notion that will have to be corrected later, and, apparently for some children, with great difficulty.

Procedures of the sort that initiate the child into the mystique of reading by drawing his attention to the visual configuration ("remember this shape; it has a tail") and its associated meaning ("the one with the tail means monkey"), without alerting him to the relevance of the phonemic structure of the word, may be sufficient for some children. Somehow, these children abstract the alphabetic principle on their own. For too many others, however, such procedures, which emphasize meaning at the outset without instruction in how an alphabet works, lead into a blind alley. The ability of the child to memorize the shapes and associated meanings of a handful of words may lull him at first into the comforting belief that he can read, but then leave him stranded at that stage—a functional illiterate with no keys to unlock new words.

What is needed is an instructional sequence that will unlock the alphabetic cipher and the world of reading for the large proportion of school children who are not learning to read by our present procedures. The same instructional sequence can be used for the quick learners as well, provided a few general principles of instruction are followed.

General Principles of Instruction

There are several interrelated principles, applicable to all classroom instruction, that are, in our view, particularly critical for successful reading acquisition. These principles are not original with us; indeed, they are probably as old as teaching itself. However, we believe they should be emphasized at the outset because, in reading instruction in our schools, they tend to be honored more often in the breach than in the observance. Ironically enough, they are typically brought into play during remedial instruction after the child has failed. The child is then said to have been resistant to ordinary methods of instruction. We suspect that if the ordinary methods of instruction had been based on these principles, the children would have been considerably less resistant. We should add that what follows is only a brief sketch of the general principles to be considered. An exhaustive treatment of the subject would require a position paper of its own.

The *first principle* is that essential skills should be taught as directly as possible with clear explanations of what is being taught. The child should not be expected to develop fundamental skills on his own by a discovery method. Though some children undoubtedly can do so, too many will fail. Those who learn quickly need not be penalized for their early success as might be feared; at the same time, the ones who have difficulty will be given a chance to acquire the information they need. This will be true, however, only if a *second principle* is observed: all procedures must be individually tailored in such a way that no child need linger at a given step after he has mastered it. This brings us to a *third principle,* the need for mastery. By mastery, we mean a high level of accuracy in the skill being taught. Too often in present day practice, a fundamental skill is introduced almost casually in one or two pages of a workbook and followed similarly by a series of additional skills in rapid succession. Instead, the understanding that is needed should be developed through as much practice and reinforcement as is required for that particular child, and all new material in a skill sequence should be preceded by a review of what has already been learned. An important *corollary of the mastery principle* is that of automatization. Mastery can imply accurate performance without regard to rate. In reading, accuracy is not enough. The accurate, but slow reader is at a considerable disadvantage. Therefore, effort should be directed toward making component skills as automatic as possible. As in all learning, practice is the key to automatization in reading acquisition.

Preparing the Child for the Alphabet

Teaching a child how to use an alphabetic system to its fullest advantage is complicated by the difficulty young children have in explicitly understanding the phonemic structure of speech. As we have said, phonemic analysis is hard because of the encodedness of spoken speech into units of syllabic size, while syllabic segmentation is much easier. However, it need not follow that the phonemic level of analysis should be bypassed entirely in favor of the syllable or the word. Instead, the child can be given a better preparation for abstracting phoneme segments both before and during reading instruction.

WORD PLAY IN EARLY CHILDHOOD

For many children, the groundwork for this difficult level of analysis begins at home before the child is old enough to go to school. Ideally, it should be extended to all preschoolers. A proper foundation laid at this time can be built upon in the prereading stages of kindergarten and at each succeeding stage of reading acquisition. Word games in early childhood that draw the child's attention to the segmental nature of his spoken language and that give him extended practice are therefore recommended. Examples of such word play include the learning of nursery rhymes and the introduction of rhyming games that use both real words and nonsense syllables. Rhyming activity makes few semantic or syntactic demands on the child while giving him practice in varying the phonemic content of utterances.

PREREADING TECHNIQUES

When the child reaches kindergarten, prereading techniques can be initiated that stress the structure of the spoken language before the instruction in the alphabet is begun. Since the word and the syllable are more readily abstracted than the phoneme, these are the structural elements of choice to introduce the child to the notion of listening for component parts of the speech stream.

Segmenting the word and the syllable. To make the *word* explicit for the child, a counting game suggested by Engelmann[41] would be useful. In this game, the teacher presents simple statements orally (for example, "John is happy"), which the child repeats. Then she says the statement again, pausing between each word, and demonstrating how to represent the number of words concretely by raising her fingers, by making chalk slashes on the board, or by using blocks as counters. The sentences can be made increasingly complex by including modifiers and function words.

Once the child understands by this method or others that the stream of speech contains word elements, the teacher can introduce the idea that the words themselves are composed of smaller units, the *syllables*. Compound words are useful at this stage of instruction (for example, "Say cowboy without the cow"), as recommended by Rosner.[33] Syllabic segmentation can be further developed with other multisyllabic words. In this case, the teacher might say the word first at a natural rate, then with short pauses between the syllables. The children are asked to repeat it after her in the same way.

Segmenting the phoneme. Instruction in abstracting segments at the level of the word and the syllable presents few problems. The word and syllable share a common characteristic—both of these segments can be separated from the speech stream with little damage to their identity as units. The teacher can accomplish this separation, as we have said, simply by pronouncing the segments individually with pauses between them. The encoded nature of the phoneme makes this kind of artificial separation of the unit more difficult.

Teacher-devised listening games can nonetheless be used to good effect in teaching phonemic segmentation. Too often in our kindergartens, they are haphazardly organized, concentrating on the initial consonants of words, and paying only scant attention to the phonemes in medial and final positions. But when they are appropriately sequenced, they can be very successful. In one such program,* a kindergarten teacher initiated prereading instruction by first teaching the children to listen for the five short vowel sounds in words. Among the games she described is one which seems particularly useful. In the first stage of the game, the teacher says a given vowel sound once ("ă"), twice ("ă ă"), or three times ("ă ă ă") and asks the class in each case to raise as many fingers as sound they have heard. After the children can do this correctly with all the short vowel sounds, she adds a final consonant to the vowel, thus producing vowel-consonant (VC) syllables ("am, it, op"). She intersperses these syllables with single phonemes of the previous lesson and again asks for finger raising. She then progresses to consonant-vowel (CV) syllables, then to CVC, CCVC, and so on, varying vowels and consonants at each stage as needed. Howard reported that after instituting this speech analysis program in the Fall, she could begin teaching reading much earlier and with greater success than ever before.[42]

The Elkonin procedure. Several auditory training programs that emphasize the analysis of syllables into phonemes (rather than the discrimination of nonspeech sounds) have been available commercially for some time. *Auditory Discrimination in Depth* is an example of this type of program.[43] None, to our knowledge, has as many worthwhile features as that outlined by the Soviet psychologist, Elkonin (Fig. 10-1).[28]

In the procedure described by Elkonin, the child is presented with a line drawing of an object which reliably elicits a word in the child's active vocabulary. Below the picture is a rectangle divided into sections equivalent to the number of phonemes in the pictured word. The child is taught to say the word slowly, putting a counter into the appropriate section of the diagram as the word is pronounced. After this game has been played with many different pictured words and the child can do the task successfully without the diagram, the idea of vowel and consonant sounds is introduced. At this time, the color of the counter is differentiated for the two phonetic classes; say—pink for the vowels and white for the consonants. Having first been taught the difference

*Marion Howard, Horace Mann School, New York, N.Y.

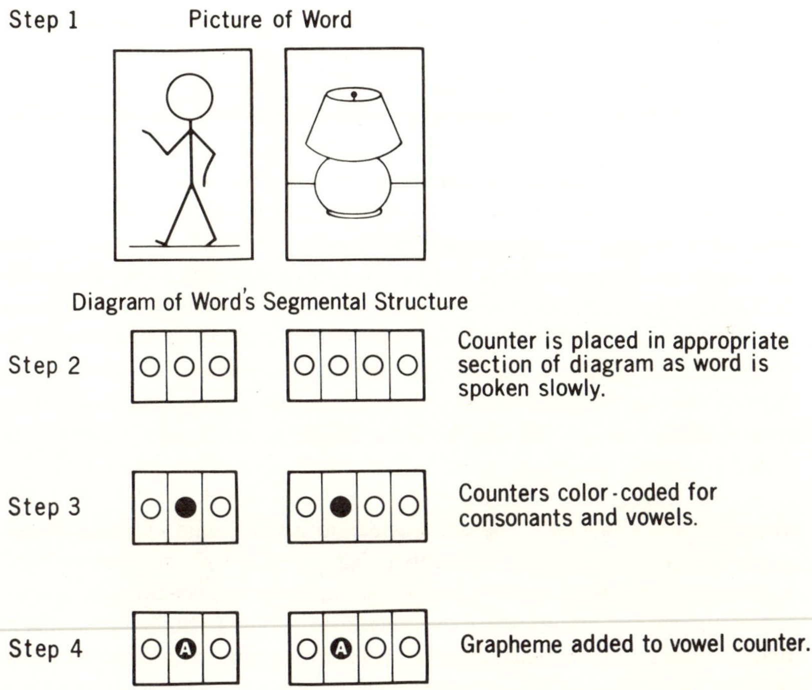

Fig. 1. This diagram is designed to facilitate analysis of the spoken word. Color-coded counters indicate consonant and vowel segments. This illustrates an adaptation of the Elkonin procedure described in the text.

between these when only one vowel is present, the child is asked to put down a pink counter whenever he hears that sound. Not before success has been attained with the five short vowel sounds is the graphic form corresponding to the sound introduced.

The Elkonin procedure has many pedagogic virtues. First, the line drawing keeps the whole word in front of the child throughout the process of analysis, obviating the need to rely on auditory memory to retain the word being studied. Second, the diagram provides a linear visual-spatial structure to which the child can relate the auditory-temporal sequence of the spoken word, thereby reinforcing the key idea of the successive segmentation of the phonemic components of the word. Third, the sections of the diagram call attention to the actual number of segments in the word, so that the child does not need to resort to uninformed guessing. Fourth, the combination of drawing, diagram, and counters provides concrete materials that help to objectify the abstract ideas being presented. Fifth, the procedure affords the child an active part to play thoughout. Finally, the color coding of the counters leads the child to appreciate the difference between vowels and consonants early in his schooling.

The actual content of the Elkonin procedure can, of course, be varied to fit the needs of a particular child or group of children. Thus it can be used not only for kindergarteners but also as a remedial technique for older children. The teacher can, for example, select for analysis syllables that contain the particular phonemes in the particular sequence deemed appropriate.

Three general rules are suggested for the selection of syllables to be segmented. First, for this early training period, the noise portion of a fricative like 's' or the nasal murmur of 'n' or 'm' would be the consonants of choice for the prevocalic position in the syllables to be analyzed. Fricatives and nasals have the advantage that, unlike other consonants (particularly the stops—'b, d, g, p, t, k'), they can be produced in isolation. They can, therefore, be used to acquaint the child with the general idea of word analysis without undue interference from coarticulation.* Second, since two-segment analysis is easier than three-segment,[32] training in segmentation might start with syllables containing two phonemes. Finally, pilot data suggest that VC syllables are easier to analyze than CV, and that both are (as we have said) easier than CVC syllables.[34] Therefore, a progression from VC to CV to CVC, in segmentation training, would probably be most efficacious.

Another approach to training in phonologic analysis is the elision technique outlined by Rosner[33] in his auditory skills program. This approach places a somewhat greater conceptual burden on the child, but could profitably be used in conjunction with the Elkonin procedure. It is always useful to offer a variety of different methods for attaining the same goals, provided that the emphasis in the auditory training is firmly placed on the analysis of the sounds of speech. Training in nonspeech sounds, which are processed quite differently, cannot be expected to have the same effect.[1]

Once the child has been taught, by whatever method, to segment spoken syllables into their phonemic components, the graphic representations of the phonemes can be introduced. The Elkonin technique of adding the letter form to the blank counters might be adopted for teaching the graphic representation of the short vowels and one or two consonants. Thereafter, it would probably be preferable to shift to a more direct procedure for teaching the letters and their phonemic equivalents. This is the stage at which the child progresses from the prereading phase to actual reading instruction.

*Coarticulation refers to the fact that the encoded consonants ('b, d, g, p, t, k', for example) cannot be produced in isolation; they are "coarticulated" with a vowel.

Basic Procedures for Initial Reading Instruction

We believe that the primary emphasis in teaching children to read in an alphabetic system should be on mapping the components of the printed word to those of the spoken word. This analytic conversion from print to speech is best accomplished, in our view, by a method that presents reading, phonics, spelling, and handwriting in coordination with each other so that instruction in each of these skills reinforces and illuminates all the others. The integration of these four aspects of alphabetic communication serves to inform the child that they are different facets of the same process and not separate, unrelated skills.

THE FIRST STEP: LETTER NAMES AND SOUNDS

We would begin reading instruction, as many so-called phonics programs do, by teaching the child to associate the shape of the letter with its name and the sound it makes. We have come to agree with Mathews[44] in his appraisal of this crucial first step:

> No matter how a child is taught to read, he comes sooner or later to the strait gate and the narrow way: he has to learn letters and the sounds for which they stand. There is no evidence whatever that he will ultimately do this better from at first not doing it all. [p. 208]

The simplest and most efficient way of teaching the sound-symbol correspondences is by the direct teaching of paired associates. The child should not be expected to abstract the correspondences for himself by a discovery method. Useful materials for teaching the alphabet are alphabet cards that include not only the upper and lower case form of the letter, but also the mnemonic of a pictured key word beginning with the sound of the letter.[45] On presentation of the card, the child is trained to recite the name of the letter, its key word, and its sound (*a*, 'apple', 'ă'). As the child learns each vowel, its symbol should be listed in a vertical column on the blackboard and reviewed each day. After the child has learned one short vowel in this way, a few consonant symbols are introduced. The remaining vowels and consonants can be taught by the same procedure in tandem with the next step. Meanwhile, the child is taught to write the same letters that he has learned to identify, not an unrelated series of letters presented in a separate writing lesson. These letters can also be incorporated into the step of the Elkonin program in which individual sounds are given graphic representations.

RELATING SPEECH TO PRINT

The next step in most reading programs that emphasize phonics would probably be "sound blending." Since letter-to-sound correspondences have been learned in isolation, the traditional phonics method requires that these be combined or blended to form words. Here the method runs afoul of the important fact about speech we have emphasized earlier: the spoken word is not a concatenated string of consecutive sounds. In speech, information about the three segments of the word 'cat' is encoded (that is, overlappingly merged) into a single sound, the syllable. Therefore, no matter how fast the consecutive phonemes are spoken, 'kŭh-ă-tŭh' abutted together consecutively will produce only the nonsense trisyllable 'kŭhătŭh' and not the monosyllabic word 'cat'.[1,5]

How can we get around the problem of the fusion of phonemes by coarticulation? Although she also uses the more traditional blending method, Slingerland (Fig. 10-2)[45] describes another technique that solves this problem fairly well. It is a spelling procedure that goes from speech to print, building on skills that have been learned in the prereading program. Instead of demanding that the child perform the impossible task of blending 'hŭh-ă-mm' to produce 'ham', the teacher first says the word 'ham', slowly, emphasizing the medial vowel. The child repeats the word, listens for the vowel sound, selects its letter card (color coded, if still necessary to help the child differentiate vowels from consonants) from a wall pocket-chart, and places it in a lower tier of the pocket-chart. The teacher then repeats the whole word and asks the child for the initial sound in the word. The child then is directed to

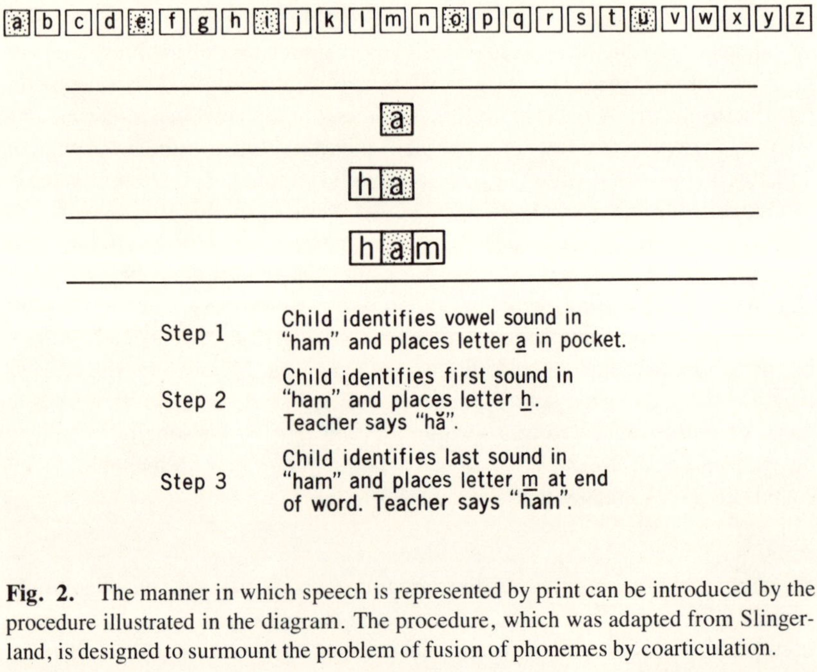

Fig. 2. The manner in which speech is represented by print can be introduced by the procedure illustrated in the diagram. The procedure, which was adapted from Slingerland, is designed to surmount the problem of fusion of phonemes by coarticulation.

pick out the appropriate letter card, identify it, and place it in front of the vowel ("Where does it go? Before the *a*, because it's the *first* sound we hear."). The teacher then draws her finger along the two letters that the child has placed in the lower tier and says: "Now we have made 'hă'. Let's listen to our word again. Our word is 'ham' (drawing out the sounds). What is the *last* sound we hear in 'ham'? That's right, it's 'mm'. Find the letter that makes the 'mm' sound. Where do we put the *m?* At the end of the word, because it's the last sound we hear." The lesson continues with the child reading aloud the whole word that has just been constructed, and ends with the child writing the word either on the blackboard or at the desk, and reading it back after it is written.

Another procedure that should be helpful in relating speech to print comes from Belgrade.[46] The teacher pronounces the sound of the initial consonant (always a nasal or fricative in the early lessons) of a simple CVC word, and writes its letter on the blackboard with a line following it. Drawing out the spoken sound for varying periods of time, the teacher shortens or lengthens the line following the letter ("s-----------, s----, s------") as appropriate. This exercise is repeated with the vowel ("ă-------, ă--------------, ă----"). Then both sounds are spoken and the interval between them varied and represented accordingly ("s-------, ă----------, s--ă---------, să---"). A consonant in final position is then added ("să-----t") and the word is spoken as a whole ("sat"). Finally, the word is written without the lines and read aloud. In subsequent lessons, the child is taught to read and write other words by the same procedure. After mastering a word, the child writes it in a notebook and perhaps uses it in a written sentence which is then read aloud. In this way, reading, writing, and spelling exercises are always coordinated, as we have also proposed. These and similar procedures[41] make concrete for the child a key fact about writing that is difficult to explain in the abstract: that the temporal succession of the overlapping and nondiscrete speech segments (the phonemes) is represented spatially by a left-to-right linear succession of discrete characters (the letters).

Thus far, the child has learned the letters and their sounds in isolation and has been taught, without using questionable blending methods, the basics of how to convert speech to sequences of letters; that is, the child has learned how to analyze the spoken word and to construct its written model. It remains to teach him how to go from print to speech.

LEARNING THE SYLLABLE TYPES OF ENGLISH

This step is probably the most critical one. It should prepare the child to make the conversion from any printed word to speech, which is what early reading acquisition is all about. A sequence of syllable presentations similar to the Hay-Wingo Ladder[47] devised by two learning disability specialists,

(Nancy Chapel and Cynthia Conway),[48] has been highly successful at this stage of reading instruction (Fig. 10-3). This sequence can be best characterized as a modification of the linguistic method of minimal contrasts, in which the unit under study is the syllable. The goal is to make the conversion from printed syllables to speech more nearly automatic by circumventing the letter-by-letter sound-out and blending of the phonics method. The procedure differs from other syllabic methods in being designed to elucidate for the child the internal construction of the syllable.

In the Chapel-Conway lessons, the short vowels are listed on the blackboard in a vertical column and reviewed, just as they had been during the alphabet drills. This time, however, a dash is added after each letter ('ă_, ĕ_, ĭ_, ŏ_, ŭ_'). The child is taught that the short vowel is always followed by a consonant, and that the dash represents a missing consonant that will be filled in later. He is then taught the game of adding a letter in front of the short vowel and pronouncing the resultant combination ('mă_, mĕ_, mĭ_, mŏ_, mŭ_'). The prevocalic consonant is then varied ('să_, sĕ_, sĭ_, sŏ_, sŭ_'). Meanwhile, the children are encouraged to think of words beginning with those syllables, and are taught to fill in the missing final consonants in those words ('man', 'met', 'mop'). The lessons continue with the addition of consonant blends to the front of the vowel ('smă_, smĕ_, smĭ_').

Step 1 Short Vowel followed by Dash
ă-
ĭ-
ŏ-
ĕ-
ŭ-

Step 2 Addition of Prevocalic Consonant
mă-
mĭ-
mŏ-
mĕ-
mŭ-

Step 3 Construction of CVC Words
măt
mĭx
mŏm
mĕn
mŭm

Step 4 Substitution of Prevocalic Consonant
să-
sĭ-
etc.

Step 5 Same as Step 3

Step 6 Substitution of Consonant Blends
smă-
smĭ-
etc.

Step 7 Construction of CCVC(C) Words
smăck
smĕll
etc.

Step 8 Vowel-e
a-e
e-e
i-e
etc.

Step 9 Construction of CVCe Words
mate
mite

Fig. 3. The chart shows a step-wise sequence of syllable presentations designed to facilitate automatic conversion from the printed word to speech. It is an adaptation of a procedure designed by Chapel and Conway, as described in the text.

When the short vowel, closed syllable has been mastered, the idea of the long vowel is introduced, again with a structured model (*a-e*). It is pointed out that the missing letter in the model is now followed by an *e*, which is silent but marks the long vowel. Games of word construction with this model are then added. In the last stage, the child learns that when these consonant-vowel combinations appear alone without the added consonant (the dash representing the missing letter is now erased), the vowel is long and matches the letter name, producing an open syllable.

The child now has at his command a number of the major elements needed for decoding phonetically-regular words. The basic contrast between the short and long vowels has been clarified, and the child has been introduced to closed, open, and silent-*e* syllables.

There remain only three phonetically-regular syllable types to be taught: the vowel team (CVVC), vowel = *r* (CV = *r*), and consonant-*le* (C = *le*) syllables. These essentially complete the child's understanding of regular syllable types and provide the basis for analysis of multisyllabic words.

SYLLABIFICATION NOW EASILY TAUGHT

Once the six basic syllable types have been mastered, syllabification is more easily understood. What the child needs to know at this stage can be described by six basic rules. These are (1) divide a compound word between the two words (hot/dog); (2) when the initial vowel is followed by two consonants, divide the word between them (muf/fin, vel/vet); (3) when the initial vowel is followed by one consonant, alternative pronunciations must be matched to words in the child's lexicon (pu/pil, lem/on); (4) when a word ends in *le*, the consonant preceding the *le* begins the last syllable (ta/ble); (5) consonant blends and digraphs are not divided when separating a word into syllables; (6) prefixes and suffixes form separate syllables (re/peat/ing).[49]

IRREGULAR WORDS

Throughout this chapter we have stressed the importance of language analysis skills needed to decode phonetically regular words. Obviously, there are words in English for which such skills are not sufficient. Among them are the small function words that are needed as soon as the child begins to read sentences. Therefore, it is essential that a few of these words be taught early in the child's reading program. Simple flashcard drills seem to be sufficient to teach them to most children; some may need a more intensive approach such as trace/copy/writing-from-memory procedures.[45]

WHICH READING TEXT SERIES TO USE

At this point, something must be said about children's readers. For many children who receive the language analysis skills approach we have outlined, one reading series will probably do about as well as another. However, for the substantial number of children who have difficulty learning to read, careful control of the linguistic progression in the vocabulary of the reading series is likely to be important for the end result. Therefore, we would recommend that instruction in language analysis skills should be followed by placement in one of the many commercially-prepared linguistic readers in which phonetically regular word patterns are presented systematically. As the skills are introduced in teacher-directed lessons, the linguistic readers will provide the child who needs it with ample opportunity to practice with a reading text composed primarily of phonetically regular words.

It is surely not happenstance that since the pioneering work of Orton,[50] most specialists who have developed remedial procedures for the reading disabled have emphasized a systematic presentation of phonetically regular word patterns.[41, 45, 51-54] However, it should not be necessary to wait until a child has failed before instituting this type of program. Initial reading instruction should emphasize from the beginning that we have an alphabetic, not an ideographic, orthography.

A Postscript on Remediation

Although we have discussed all of the above procedures in terms of regular classroom instruction, these same techniques are the mainstays of remedial programs. Many of the children in need of remedial instruction do not understand the intimate relationship between speech and the orthography. It is of utmost importance that we make this link explicit for them. However, since these children are frequently older and have experienced years of school failure, their needs differ from the six-year-old entering school. Many of the procedures described previously must be adapted to suit the older child. For example, the language analysis activities preliminary to reading instruction can be carried out with words from an age-appropriate vocabulary, colloquial words or nonsense syllables.

Motivating these children for the actual reading task often requires the use of materials relevant to their experiences. An excellent example of this for the older teenager is the use of the Driver's Manual as the core reading text. The phonetically regular and irregular words to be studied can be extracted directly from the manual, their selection determined by needs disclosed in the prior testing. The regular words from the manual can be used to illustrate the basic syllable types, and the others taught as sight words. The language-experience approach, wherein the students compose their own reading material, can be used in an analogous fashion. Additional practice of the phonic generalizations with nonsense syllables ensures that the child can apply the rules to decode new words.

A recently devised remedial program, *The GFB Perceptual Training Drills,*[51] contains several desirable components. Accuracy word lists are used to measure mastery of the six basic syllable types. The suggested sequence enables the student to read multisyllable words early in the program, a highly motivating factor for older students. Once a skill (for example, closed syllables with short 'ă') is mastered, speed drills are intoduced to help bring this skill to an automatic level. Also included is a list of frequently used irregular words, as well as flash cards for teaching sound-symbol relationships. Charts are provided with each component for recording individual progress. This visual representation of progress is especially motivating to the child who has experienced failure in school.

REFERENCES

1. Liberman IY: Basic research in speech and lateralization of language: Some implications for reading disability. Bull Orton Soc 21:71–87, 1971
2. Liberman IY, Shankweiler D: Speech, the alphabet, and teaching to read, in Resnick LB, Weaver PA (eds): Theory and Practice of Early Reading. vol II Hillsdale, New Jersey, Erlbaum Associates, 1979
3. Eimas PD, Siqueland ER, Juscyk P, Vigorito, J: Speech perception in infants. Science 171:303–306, 1971
4. Furth H: Thinking Without Language: Psychological Implications of Deafness. New York, The Free Press, 1966
5. Liberman AM, Cooper FS, Shankweiler D, Studdert-Kennedy M: Perception of the speech code. Psychol Rev 74:431–461, 1967
6. Liberman IY, Shankweiler D, Fischer FW, Carter B: Explicit syllable and phoneme segmentation in the young child. J Exp Child Psychol 18:201–212, 1974
7. Diringer D: The Alphabet. New York, Philosophical Library, 1948
8. Gelb IJ: A Study of Writing. Chicago, University of Chicago Press, 1963
9. Liberman IY: Segmentation of the spoken word and reading acquisition. Bull Orton Soc 23:65–77, 1973
10. Liberman IY, Shankweiler D, Liberman AM, Fowler C, Fischer FW: Phonetic segmentation and recoding in the beginning reader, in Reber AS, Scarborough D (eds): Reading: Theory and Practice. Hillsdale, New Jersey, Erlbaum Associates, 1977
11. Shankweiler D, Liberman IY: Exploring the relations between reading and speech, in Knights RM, Bakker DJ (eds): Neuropsychology of Learning Disorders: Theoretical Approaches. Baltimore, University Park Press, 1976
12. Polanyi M: Personal Knowledge: Towards a Post-critical Philosophy. New York, Harper & Row, 1964
13. Monroe M: Children Who Cannot Read. Chicago, University of Chicago Press, 1932
14. Savin HB: What the child knows about speech when he starts to learn to read, in Kavanagh JF, Mattingly IG (eds): Language by Ear and by Eye: The Relationships Between Speech and Reading. Cambridge, M.I.T. Press, 1972
15. Johnson D, Myklebust H: Learning Disabilities. New York, Grune & Stratton, 1967
16. Fant CGM: Descriptive analysis of the acoustic aspects of speech. Logos 5:3–17, 1962

17. Stevens KN: Segments, features, and analysis by synthesis, in Kavanagh JF, Mattingly IG (eds): Langauge by Ear and By Eye: The Relationships Between Speech and Reading. Cambridge, M.I.T. Press, 1972
18. Liberman AM: The grammars of speech and language. Cognitive Psychol 1:301–323, 1970
19. Fletcher H: Speech and Hearing. New York, Van Nostrand, 1929
20. Makita K: The rarity of reading disability in Japanese children. Am J Orthopsychiatry, 38:599–614, 1968
21. Rozin P, Poritsky S, Sotsky R: American children with reading problems can easily learn to read English represented by Chinese characters. Science 171:1264–1267, 1971
22. Bruce LJ: The analysis of word sounds by young children. Br J Educ Psychol 34:158–170, 1964
23. Goldstein DM: Learning to read and developmental changes in covert speech in a word analysis and synthesis skill. Unpublished Ph.D. dissertation, University of Connecticut, 1974
24. Rosner J, Simon DP: The auditory analysis test: An initial report. J Learn Disabil 4:40–48, 1971
25. Bloomfield L: Linguistics and reading. Elementary English 18:125–130; 183–186, 1942
26. Calfee R, Chapman R, Venezky R: How a child needs to think to learn to read, in Gregg LW (ed): Cognition in Learning and Memory. New York, John Wiley and Sons, 1972
27. Downing J: Comparative Reading. New York, Macmillan, 1973
28. Elkonin DB: U.S.S.R., in Downing J (ed): Comparative Reading. New York, Macmillan, 1973
29. Gibson EJ, Levin H: The Psychology of Reading. Cambridge, M.I.T. Press, 1975
30. Gleitman LR, Rozin P: Teaching reading by use of a syllabary. Reading Res Q 8:447–483, 1973
31. Vellutino FR: Alternative conceptualizations of dyslexia: Evidence in support of a verbal-deficit hypothesis. Harvard Educ Rev 47:334–354, 1977
32. Helfgott J: Phonemic segmentation and blending skills of kindergarten children: Implications for beginning reading acquisition. Contemp Educ Psychol 1:157–169, 1976
33. Rosner J: Helping Children Overcome Learning Disabilities. New York, Walker & Company, 1975
34. Treiman RA: Children's ability to segment speech into syllables and phonemes as related to their reading ability. Unpublished manuscript, Department of Psychology, Yale University, 1976
35. Zifcak M: Phonological awareness and reading acquisition in first grade children. Unpublished Ph.D. dissertation, University of Connecticut, 1977
36. Fowler CA, Liberman IY, Shankweiler D: On interpreting the error pattern in beginning reading. Lang Speech 20:162–173, 1977
37. Shankweiler D, Liberman IY: Misreading: A search for causes, in Kavanagh JF, Mattingly IG (eds): Language By Ear and By Eye: The Relationships Between Speech and Reading. Cambridge, M.I.T. Press, 1972
38. Daniels JC, Diack H: Progress in Reading. Nottingham, University of Nottingham Institute of Education, 1956
39. Weber R: A linguistic analysis of first-grade errors: A survey of the literature. Read Res Q 4:96–119, 1970
40. Venezky RL: Discussion, in Kavanagh JF (ed): Communicating by Language: The Reading Process. Bethesda, National Institute of Child Health and Human Development, 1968
41. Engelmann S: Preventing Failure in the Primary Grades. Chicago, Science Research Associates, 1969
42. Howard M: Personal communication, April 5, 1974

43. Lindamood CH, Lindamood PC: Auditory Discrimination in Depth. Boston, Teaching Resources, 1969
44. Mathews M: Teaching to Read Historically Considered. Chicago, University of Chicago Press, 1966
45. Slingerland BH: A Multi-sensory Approach to Language Arts for Specific Language Disability Children: A Guide for Primary Teachers. Cambridge, Educators Publishing Service, 1971
46. Vladisavljevic S: Personal communication, June 2, 1976
47. Hay J, Wingo C: Reading with Phonics, Philadelphia, Lippincott, 1960
48. Chapel N, Conway C: Personal communication, March 10, 1976
49. Lerner JW: Children With Learning Disabilities. Boston, Houghton Mifflin, 1971
50. Orton ST: Word-blindness in school children. Arch Neurol Psychiatry 14:581–615, 1925
51. Gallistel E, Fischer P, Blackburn M: GFB Perceptual Training Drills for Teaching Reading and Spelling in the Concept Transfer Sequence. New Haven, Montage Press, 1974
52. Gillingham A, Stillman B: Remedial Training for Children with Specific Reading Disability in Reading, Spelling, and Penmanship. Cambridge, Educators Publishing Service, 1960
53. Schmerler F: The Schmerler Instructional Sequence and Strategies for Reading and Spelling. St. Paul, EMC Corporation, 1973
54. Spaulding R, Spaulding W: The Writing Road to Reading. New York, Whiteside & Morrow, 1957
55. Morais J, Cary L, Alegria J, Bertelson P: Does awareness of speech as a sequence of phones arise spontaneously? Cognition 7:323–331, 1979
56. Lukatela G, Turvey M: Some experiments on the Roman and Cyrillic alphabets of Serbo-Croatian, in Kavanagh JF, Venezky RL (eds): Orthography, Reading, and Dyslexia. Baltimore, University Park Press, 1980

Subject Index

a b c d e f g h i j
0 1 2
8